The Healing Bee

by

Roch Domerego

Translated by Francine Sagar

First English Edition
NORTHERN BEE BOOKS
2016

THE HEALING BEE by Roch Domerego.
Translated by Francine Sagar.

All rights reserved. No part of this publication may be reproduced, stored in a retrieval system, transmitted in any form or by any means electronic, mechanical, including photo-copying, recording or otherwise without prior consent of the copyright holders.

The publishers are not responsible for the medical advice given in this volume.

First English Edition Published in 2016 by Northern Bee Books
Scout Bottom Farm
Mytholmroyd
Hebden Bridge, HX7 5JS.

www.northernbeebooks.co.uk
Tel: 01422 882751

ISBN: 978-1-908904-84-3

For my daughter Anastasia.

In order to hand over our planet just as you entrusted it to me.

Index

1. The Power of the Honeybee..9

2. A Child from the South..13

3. Honey for Hope...27

4. African Magic 43

5. The Invisible Medicine 55

6. Apitherapy 61

7. The Humanitarian Solution..77

8. Soldiering On...95

9. A Pharmacopeia Direct from the Hive.............................109

10. Medicine from the Honeybees...131

11. Therapeutic Usage of Products from the Hive................137

Alphabetical Listing of Ailments...141

1. The Power of the Honeybee

What if the bee were to be man's oldest friend? This is an absurd suggestion for the vast majority of people, who tend to lump together – and to fear intrinsically – all insects that carry a venomous sting; this old fear of 'the other' takes many forms. Yet, a honeybee will never come and forage on your dinner plate in the way of her carnivorous cousin the wasp. The honeybee's dreaded sting is not an offensive weapon. It is merely a means of self-defence and, moreover, it is a suicidal act for the bee. You only have to observe honeybees for a few minutes to realise that, unlike the much more dangerous mosquitoes, these peaceful creatures are not in the least bit interested in our delicate skin; honeybees are, with the exception of the silkworm, the only insects that man has ever managed to domesticate, thereby profiting immensely.

You can come to like honeybees, and you can get them to like you; I would even go as far as saying that to like them is a duty. Ancient civilizations had understood this, and today all over the world there are many of us who share this conviction. All you have to do is make time to get to know the bees. You then enter an extraordinary, fascinating and boundless universe where resources are unlimited, both from the physical and the spiritual points of view.

The cathedral builders of yesteryear never left anything to chance. Even down to every subliminal detail, everything was engineered to condition whoever entered God's house. The faithful had to be made to feel His presence, often to the point of metaphorically being crushed under His power. It was a case of acting upon peoples' senses in order to impress their minds.

A hive is like a living cathedral. You should only approach it with humility. If you are not in the right frame of mind, punishment is immediately forthcoming. Like many other animals, honeybees can sense fear, or aggressiveness, in whoever enters their territory, and they react accordingly. If you believe that the bees are going to attack, you are certain to get stung. If you anticipate venom to be pain-inducing, you are guaranteed to feel pain. By contrast, if you approach the hive with confidence and with an open heart, if you show the bees love and respect, you will be welcomed as a friend, and not treated as a trespasser. You will then discover that to be given the immense privilege of communicating or even communing with the colony brings forth feelings of well-being of a rare intensity. When you take part in the bees' harmonious life, you gain access to a near-perfect world and you can find your own equilibrium.

Thanks to its nice taste, people are ready to admit to the possibility that honey might be "good for your health", but people also have an irrational fear of venom, which is perceived as an evil poison. Wrongly, as it turns out, since venom can also bring along its share of beneficial effects. Perhaps we can explain this dread by going back to another animal that haunts the Christian world's collective unconscious: the snake from the garden of Eden.

Yet the snake is also a creature with two sides, and the Aztecs had no hesitation in worshipping it by adorning it with feathers from birds. From India to the Mediterranean, the snake is associated with the art of healing. Hermes, messenger of the gods, leader of souls and master of magic and alchemy, had for his principal emblem the Caduceus, made from a laurel or olivetree branch, surmounted by a pair of wings and encircled by two intertwined snakes; this has a strange resonance with the double helix found in DNA, to which everything always points back. Amongst Chinese Taoists, the caduceus takes on the form of yin-yang, a symbol of two entwined and complimentary serpentine shapes in one androgynous and vital principle. Ever since Asclepius, or Aesculapius for the Romans, the snake appears on its own, but it remains the symbol of modern medicine. Why should we fear it?

You cannot separate honey from venom. Day and night do not oppose one another, but succeed each other and make each other whole. The unity of the honeybee is also founded on this duality. You have to love it as a whole if you are to reach into the heart of nature, to which we owe everything since the beginning of time. A long and tortuous path has been required to get from mineral to vegetal, from

1. THE POWER OF THE HONEYBEE

vegetal to animal, and then from animal to man, and we must always bear in mind that it has taken millions of years to get the wonderful things that we now have at our disposal, but that it would only take man's bad influence a few decades to destroy everything.

Honeybees are everywhere, on every continent, and occur throughout man's history - amongst the Aborigines, in Africa, in Nepal, in Babylon as well as in Madagascar, and in parts of Chinese, Inca and Egyptian civilizations. Drawings depicting honey-gathering have even been found on the walls of prehistoric caves. In Greek mythology, Artemis's high priestesses were called 'bees'. The druids in Gaul used to associate honeybees with the revered oak tree. The sacred texts – Bhagavad-gita, Koran, Old and New Testaments – all refer to the presence of bees in many instances. Archangel Gabriel, in particular, is always "surrounded by the humming of bees" whenever he appears to Mary or to Mohamed.

Bees are obviously God's messengers. They are respected and revered, which explains why many kings have adopted them as their symbol.

In Sophism, a mystical branch of Islam, honeybees are present from birth until death. Meditation takes place in front of beehives, and a drop of honey is placed under the tongue of the dead, in order to facilitate the 'passage' to the afterlife. In Morocco, where the Sophist tradition is very strong, the King, who is descended from Mohamed, is the 'keeper' of the country's bees; and the teaching of the prophet, this unique and ubiquitous creature is often referred to. "He who takes of the honey three mornings each month will be guarded against serious illness." Not only do they of course act as intermediaries between nature and man, but in whichever religion you look at, honeybees also possess boundless powers which enable us to heal our body and to guide our spirit. This, as always, represents unity within duality. Through the honeybee we find body-soul spirit equilibrium and harmony.

The day I understood this simple and blinding truth, I knew that I was lost no longer.

2. A Child from the South

I was about four years old when I first saw some beehives. I had just lost my father, whose car had crashed into a plane tree on a road in the Herault district. My mother had sent me to stay with my uncle and aunt in the Alpes-de-Haute-Provence, in order to give herself time to get over the shock and try to get organized. Her whole universe had just fallen apart. She was left with three children: my sisters were aged six and eleven.

Like many men, my father had been so absorbed in his business dealings that he had never planned for such a tragedy. He had vision and he went in for big projects: a Ford garage, a petrol station, the first car-parks in Montpellier city-centre – he was banking on building a future. He lost. Life is a relentless gamble that can strip you of everything in a flash. After fifteen years of never-ending and exhausting legal wrangling, my mother was left with nothing of what her husband had tried to build.

I can barely remember my first stay at Les Mées, a little town halfway between Sisteron and Forcalquier, nestled at the foot of enormous rocks nicknamed the Penitents; legend has it that they are in fact the bodies of travellers turned into stone by the queen of Provence, because one of them had committed the sacrilege of looking at her whilst she was bathing naked in the Durance river. It is a grandiose site, imbued with a certain sadness, which has always mirrored the state of mind I found myself in. I recall my days as being lulled by the incessant buzzing from some fifty beehives that my aunt looked after assiduously – and that I wasn't allowed to approach under any pretext.

"If you get married again, you will cease to exist!" That was the judgement that my uncle, my father's brother, had one day passed on my poor mother. It would take a long time before the notion of women's liberation, which was all the rage amongst Paris intellectuals, would reach as far as our provincial areas.

By the time I was old enough to go to secondary school, my mother didn't feel strong enough to carry on raising a boy without the support of a man. She didn't know how to go about it. That is when, as suggested by my uncle, she offered me the opportunity to become a boarder in Digne (we were at the time living in a council flat in Nice); from there I would easily be able to spend the weekends in Les Mées, only twenty-five kilometres away. It didn't take me long to make a decision. My youngest sister was about to leave home. I was still a child and had nothing in common with the eldest, now aged twenty two. Ever since the accident, my mother had been living in a parallel universe. Despite my having proclaimed myself 'man of the house', I was glad to leave, not only in order to relieve her, but also because I secretly aspired to discover another world. I wasn't going to be disappointed.

In Digne, the Lycée Gassendi had a reputation as one of the toughest in France, and that title was well deserved. The deputy head was an ex-legionnaire from Corsica who took pride in taming the students placed under his authority and instilling in them his own implacable discipline.

It has to be said that we were no angels. My fellow students came from the surrounding area and were the sons of peasants, rough and always ready to pick a fight, with no sense of suffering. Despite my city origins, I soon established myself as the head of one of the two rival gangs; they were comprised of kids of the same age who fought over some imaginary power using fists reinforced with padlocks, just to make sure the arguments would be really hard-hitting. I became a real toughie. However, at the same time, I could feel in a confused way that I was also harbouring a positive sort of energy.

I really became aware of this as I was standing in one of the corridors, on a day when our games were a little more peaceful than usual. One boy was standing still, eyes shut, and we were playing at miming mysterious gestures around him, as though to cast a spell on him, until he would lose his balance. I was in the process of moving my hands around his face, without touching his skin, when he suddenly announced that he could "feel my hands". Without at first believing any of it, the others soon wanted to have a go, and they noticed feeling

2. A CHILD FROM THE SOUTH

the same effect. We were far too young to draw any conclusions from the incident, and I simply became known as "the wizard".

I had noticed another strange phenomenon, a very personal one this time. Every time I walked along the pavement along the wall of the orphanage in Digne, I could feel, through its open windows, such strong vibrations that I would burst into tears. It was not a form of sadness, nor was it compassion. It was a much stronger, much deeper feeling which I wasn't able to identify.

*

The four years I spent at secondary school could be described as a surprising mixture of two novels: Sans Famille, of which I still carry an old time-worn copy at the bottom of my bag, and Les Disparus de Saint-Agil. We would spend evenings hiding in the outbuildings just for the pleasure of a shared cigarette which we would pass between us with the same fervour that others, seemingly a thousand leagues from our own universe, would use to pass around a "spliff". One of the night watchmen, a benign hunchback, would pretend not to notice anything, whilst another, who was a bit on the sadistic side, would slyly tell on us. Thereby I sometimes found myself kneeling on the dormitory floor tiles, arms outstretched, for two hours, under the watchful eye of a supervisor tasked with hitting me on the hands as soon as I lowered my arms.

I was an average pupil. Except in maths, at which I excelled with what seemed to others like nauseating ease. The famous "flair" for maths! A poisoned chalice. By the second year, we were using a textbook with worksheets for individual work. By Christmas I had answered all the questions! Of course I would daydream during lessons, until one day my teacher was astonished to discover the completed workbook. This kind woman, although a good pedagogue, would never accept that I had accomplished such a workload and she accused me of having cheated. Like many children when placed in this situation, I decided to simply stop dead in my tracks. They wanted me to be a bad student. I was going to prove them right, and from now on I would only do the minimum.

I wasn't able to leave the school each weekend. In order to do that, first of all I would have had to escape the many hours of detention that I always seemed to accumulate, as though I didn't really want that freedom which I had been denied. Paradoxically, I had ended up feeling at home within the boarding school. This kind of resigned acceptance lasted quite a long time for me. All the hotels where I stayed would seem like home. Those soul-less places built to shelter passing guests would appear familiar to me.

I was not happy at my uncle's. I wasn't unhappy either. I think he had taken me in because I was his brother's son, but that he didn't really feel bound by that clannish duty. Neither he nor his wife would ever show me any real affection. They didn't know how. It wasn't their way of life. Nevertheless, they did teach me a lot, without really knowing they were doing it.

I learned about Provence during shooting or fishing expeditions reminiscent of Pagnol's novels. My uncle was a former forestry worker and an average hunter. He would merely carry a gun whilst walking his dog as the saying goes. On Sunday mornings I would follow him from a distance, my 14mm rifle in hand, but I never so much as hit a skylark. He would stop as soon as he had shot two partridges, declaring that he had to leave some for nature as well as for other hunters. Then again, he was a well-known fisherman, and would get eighty trout out of the river one after the other without tiring. He would never give advice. "Come behind me and observe." It was a true spectacle, but that was that as far as his teaching methods would stretch. However, with just a few uttered sentences he would tell me more about nature than I would have learnt in the pages of a whole encyclopaedia.

On the day of my fourteenth birthday, he decided to teach me to drive, and hoisted the car onto blocks so that I could practise going through the gears. Like all beginners, I would let out the clutch too fast and stalled the car twice in quick succession. That brought the lesson to an end, and there would never be another.

My aunt, for her part, would spend her time telling me over and over again: "Good job you're not my son!". Coming from a woman who couldn't have children, this indicated a terrifying coldness, which I could not fathom. In spite of all this, she shared with me her passion for beekeeping and she "taught me the bees". She managed the veritable tour de force of passing on to me her love of beekeeping, without giving me any love at all.

2. A CHILD FROM THE SOUTH

She had been doing this job for more than thirty years, and she was probably one of the few women in the profession. She was therefore all the more respected in the area. The experience she had acquired seemed daunting to those in this closed, semi-secret society where not all were given the right codes to get by. The first time she invited me to come along to the hives I was scared. At the beginning, a fear of getting stung completely spoils the encounter with this marvellous world. Nevertheless, as soon as I found myself in the middle of the constant and deafening humming, I immediately knew that it was familiar to me. Wearing my funny little hat with a veil attached to it, I figured I was like an explorer who had just encountered an idyllic civilization that is only too happy to welcome him. There emanated from the hives and their occupants an incredible energy that was filling me with joy. I will never forget that moment.

From Spring to Autumn I would spend the whole of my free time tending the bees. My aunt would take me along wherever she went, be it to purchase bits of kit or to sell her products, and I was proudly introduced to the inner circle of initiates. I discovered that beekeepers form a kind of large family whose members share an unlimited passion for the insect they revere. I was convinced that this 'family' would become my family. I couldn't have known then how large it would become. During their conversations I was at first surprised to hear that there was as much talk about therapy as there was about beekeeping. I had naively thought that honeybees were agricultural workers; I soon realised that they are also precious medical assistants, and that their hives are like laboratories.

In rural areas, science had not yet swept everything out of its path. People would not hesitate to go from the doctor to the bonesetter, unless they went straight to the faith healer. Without knowing it, they were merely validating the psychosomatic dimension of many ailments, the side that only heals when there is perfect trust between the patient and the person who looks after him, therefore when there is within the patient himself a certain trust in the healing process, whatever medicine is administered. It would nevertheless take official medicine a very long time before it would admit the importance of the psychological side of things.

Not that it was all about faith and magic either. Some people knew the power of plants, whose secrets had been passed from generation to generation since time immemorial, and which were just as efficient, if not more so, than any industrially produced pharmacopeia. At the time though, such practices were regarded as having only just survived from the middle ages. Who would have thought that, years later, chemists would be proud to display the words "Herbal Medicine" on their shop-fronts?

There were also some real "wise men". One of my uncle's two neighbours was a giant of a man whose sun-beaten face always peered from under a black beret, and whose hands were as big as those of a washerwoman's wooden beaters. He had received from his mother, who in turn had got it from her own mother, the gift of "taking away the fire". Like a modern-day Jesus Christ, he would sit at the bedside of someone who had received burns, and he would delicately lay his enormous hands and gnarled fingers on the burnt area, whilst muttering some sort of prayer whose words were known only to himself. Any pain would disappear instantly, and, after a few days, the wound would heal without leaving any scarring. The first time I witnessed one of these sessions, I was speechless. So, science was not able to solve everything, or to explain everything. There remained inaccessible areas of darkness amongst its universal light. I felt both disturbed and relieved.

I had a privileged relationship with this man. Where others saw magic, I had felt that there was love. It was a different sort of love, one that I had never before managed to define precisely, but that I could feel intensely when I was near him. I would later come to understand that he "shone". He had promised to pass on to me the secret of his prayer, but he passed away before I became old enough to be worthy of it.

Today when I am asked how I can explain such healings, and what power can inhabit people capable of performing such "miracles", I confess that I do not have an answer; or perhaps only a very incomplete one. A skin that has been burnt has lost its energy. Some people are gifted with the ability to "recharge" the damaged area. It has even been possible to photograph the alteration in the energy field after a laying on of hands. How, though? Here we step into the unknown.

2. A CHILD FROM THE SOUTH

I know that it is particularly difficult to admit this in the country of Descartes, but like Professor Damazio I prefer to state:- "I feel, therefore I am." Personally, I like a bit of mystery. It represents one of the facets of what Tibetan people call "impermanence", the invisible part of reality, the part that it is not possible to understand. In fact, when one day I told one of them that I was beginning to understand the meaning of "impermanence", he replied smilingly that I was lacking one element, because I was thinking within the permanent side of "impermanence" and that, beyond, there existed "the impermanence of impermanence." A lesson in humility if ever there was one.

*

Following my O'Levels, I moved to the agricultural college in Gardanne, situated between Aix-en-Provence and Marseille. Three hundred students on a five hundred hectare campus: wind, scrubland, girls, freedom… I remained very keen on maths and science, but my universe wasn't a closed one. What I had seen and experienced had taught me that nothing lasts forever. I didn't distinguish between the scientific and the irrational or between rigorous processes and emotive reactions. I used to tell myself that, given time, the impossible always remains probable, and that what matters is the acquisition of experience. It is important to move away from beliefs, which can limit your horizon. To believe is to impose limits on oneself, it means forbidding oneself to go further. No, you have to keep your senses and your mind open. Whatever the old proverb says about killing the cat, curiosity is an indispensable attribute.

I started to take advantage of the "powers" that nature had given me to alleviate pain in those suffering back problems or headaches. I was also conducting trivial experiments. One of my friends would place his cigarette lighter somewhere on the school football playing fields, and I had to guess its location by moving my pendulum across a scale drawing of the pitch. Seeing my success, the others soon encouraged me to do something more useful. Still using the pendulum, I was able to work out what would be the main topics in our forthcoming exams. I was not predicting. Let's just say that I was simply "feeling" the choice of questions, which had been prepared by the local exam boards a long time beforehand. This enabled us to better target our revision.

I would also make myself useful amongst the young university students paid to supervise us, who had heard about my reputation, and who would call upon me regarding their own deadlines. Having just passed his Geography finals, one of them got hold of me, laughing:-

- *"Come here, you, let me give you a bear hug!"*
- *"Did it turn out like I said?"*
- *"Yes, to the last comma! My paper was a real blinder."*
- *"But tell me, you had also revised the rest, just in case?"*
- *"Not at all!"*

That day I must confess that his absolute confidence did frighten me a little.

*

Upon my arrival at the college, I had been elected deputy head boy, and the plan was for me to work alongside the sixth former who would then train me as his successor. By October, following an accident which had put him in a cast for several months, I found myself in charge. As a new boy, I was proud to be suddenly given this responsibility, and the tough experiences I had been through at secondary school enabled me to perform my duties without too much difficulty.

> *"It was while I was acting in this capacity that one day a group of pupils came to ask my permission to use the amphitheatre during lunch break. The kitchen porter was a thirty-something called Hervé who was, according to them, a Kung-fu master - and they had got him to invite them along for some Kung-fu classes. Of course I acquiesced immediately and opened the room for them, stipulating that as I was in charge I would have to sit through the lessons."*

I had for a long time been attracted by martial arts. I had not read any books on the subject, and I just about knew the name Bruce Lee, having seen none of his films, but the topic was somehow anchored deep within me. For two months I sat in a corner, not saying a word, observing keenly everything that was going on down on the stage.

Two months was what it took for my nine mates to lose their enthusiasm, and one after the other they gave up when faced with the strict

2. A CHILD FROM THE SOUTH

rigour of the teaching they were being presented with. Hervé, by asking them to carry out meditation exercises before, during and at the end of lessons, had totally disconcerted them. They thought he was mad. They had come to fight, not to think.

One day, after warming up and finding that he was on his own, he turned to me:-

– *"I don't think any of them is going to turn up today."*

I stood up and walked towards him with the certitude that I was the one he was waiting for.

They will not come any more. I am the one who wants to learn. You want to learn kung-fu? You have been watching for two months. Show me what you have learnt. Here, hit me.

And as he was lifting his left arm, showing me the side of his thorax, just under the armpit, I tried very hard to make the perfect gesture and hit him gently, so as not to hurt him too much. He slapped me on the face, really hard.

– *"Hit me!"*

I was surprised by his reaction, so I hit him a second time, a bit harder this time. He feigned another slap, but it was his foot that hit me square on the buttocks with such force that even my head was left ringing.

– *"I told you to hit me!"*

I still didn't understand. For someone who had been in fights more than once without ever giving the matter a second thought, I couldn't bring myself to hit a man for whom I felt respect, and who was deliberately offering up one of the most delicate parts of the human body. I forced myself to strike for the third time, only for slaps on the face and butt kicks to rain on me like never before. Hervé looked straight into my eyes and repeated, as if it was the only word he knew:-

– *"Hit!"*

Tears were running down my cheeks. He had hurt me, physically as well as morally. Suddenly, I felt hatred towards him. I wanted to see him on the ground. I hit him as hard as I could. He lowered his arms, as if nothing had happened, and said:-

— *"You see, this is what Kung-fu is about. You have to feel it if you want to learn."*

He left the room, leaving me totally distraught. This had been my first lesson; I should have been put off for ever. The opposite happened, and I became his disciple for seven years. Four hours a day, six days a week.

This was a discipline, or I dare say an asceticism, to which my rebellious temperament would spontaneously submit. Kung-fu had found me, and I had found my master. Nevertheless, it took me three years before I dared use the word master with Hervé, who never availed himself of the title. At the beginning, noticing that I was unsure as to how to address him, he had said:- "I am me. You call me what you feel is right." He wasn't granting me a privilege, I was the one imposing a burden on him. Within the Asiatic tradition, the student chooses his master. If he fails, this only occurs because their relationship was not a harmonious one.

One speaks, the other listens; one knows and the other is learning: master thinker, schoolmaster, music teacher, project manager, master craftsman… All our modern civilizations are built on this relationship , which is not to be confused with that of master to slave, which is at the base of another model, an economic system shattered by the little revolutionary phrase "Love thy neighbour."

During those seven years, I leant to know each and every fragment of my body and to master it in order better to use its capacity. I was at the very peak of physical condition. But this wonderful "machine" is nothing without a soul. One must also learn to explore every nook and cranny of one's own brain, to control all of its emotions without suppressing any of them. One must learn to channel one's energy, and how to receive an adversary's energy in order to appropriate it and then to return it a hundred times more powerful. Mass and energy: despite appearances, we have not strayed far from Einstein. Spirit and matter form a perfect union.

2. A CHILD FROM THE SOUTH

During the first few sessions, while my master was adopting a meditation posture, I didn't know what to do, and I didn't dare question him. I would merely observe him. Should I be sitting down as he was? What should I be thinking about? I thought I was supposed to empty my head and I couldn't achieve it. Then I started to feel that on the contrary you were supposed to fill you mind with presence, with intensity. After a few months, I was able to spend whole hours in meditation, sitting on a bench on the Cours Mirabeau street, right in the heart of Aix-en-Provence, not hearing or seeing anybody.

To start with I was full of enthusiasm and I approached Hervé:-

- *"I have a lot of questions to ask you."*
- *"If there are too many questions, then we will have no questions."*

Or another time:-

- *"Today I feel really great; I'll be able to do two hundred press-ups and three hundred stomach exercises, no problems."*
- *"Right then, in that case, let's meditate."*

Sometimes, when he did answer one of my questions, I would regret having asked, because his response would raise a myriad more queries. Hervé would always smile. He was both the sword and the rock, in perfect equilibrium. He would emit a sort of intense softness, yet incredibly strong violence could spring up instantly. In order to be efficient, an attack must surprise. Kung-fu is not a combat sport but a martial art; this is a more important distinction than would appear at first glance. You don't learn to fight, you learn about death. There are of course a number of ritual gestures that need to be respected, but they are only a means to an end.

The ultimate act is to defend one's territory, that is to say one's "being", up to the total annihilation of one's designated opponent, at any cost. From the moment you decide to start a fight, you coldly accept that it will be brought to its conclusion. This is done without hatred but also without pity. The precept is simple: "If you don't kill him it means that you do not respect him."

Respect is itself a master word. If it gets ignored then fighting or even wars ensue, and that is true in all human groups, be they large or small. In the same way as a white cell destroys a bacterium in order to preserve the safety of an organism, no intruder can penetrate a beehive. Here is a perfect illustration of the notion of living space, taken at its most basic level.

To learn means to constantly question oneself, but also to cast a critical eye on the master himself in order to find one's own way. One must know that the master is not perfect, since perfection, like permanence, does not exist. If they did, how boring would the world be! Although this may appear paradoxical at first, it may well be that imperfection is the source of harmony.

Hervé and I lost touch with each other in the same way as we had met. After a last unreal fight, in the middle of the night and at the heart of a forest near Les Mées, we offered each other one last salute, and our lives went on to follow their separate paths. There always comes a time when master and pupil must part. The teaching remains.

2. A CHILD FROM THE SOUTH

3. Honey for Hope

In 1980 I had to interrupt my biology studies at Nice University, which I had entered into straight after taking the baccalaureate. The time had come when I was not allowed to postpone military service for any longer than I already had. Like most of the youths who had to comply with this obligation, I wasn't best pleased. Unlike some, however, I was not willing to attempt absolutely anything, including feigning insanity, in order to be exempted. I was perfectly willing to dedicate a year of my life to society, but I wanted this to serve a purpose.

If you merely submit to a process, you simply survive; whereas I was determined to live through it, and life is nothing without passion. Yet I also realised that in the absence of action, passion is but an illusion, or a vague impulse. Nowadays I often say that to act is like praying: "Heaven helps those who help themselves". Let's be clear however, I do not use these words in their Catholic sense. People need a goal, of whatever kind, and must give themselves the means to attain that goal. To go in search of your heart's desires is to embark on the most wonderful of journeys.

I heard about "la coopération" – a scheme by which you could do some unpaid work abroad in lieu of national service; this so-called "barefoot volunteer" scheme – the Volunteers - was a humanitarian organisation offering me the chance to do something useful whilst fulfilling my military obligations. I could be at once selfish and altruistic, helping others whilst helping myself.

Who can tell whether this was due to chance or whether it was my destiny? I never look at it in those terms; it may be that we will not find the key to such mysteries until after we are dead. What matters is to follow one's chosen path, to remain in harmony with oneself and with the universe, and with life. There is no point in swimming against the tide of one's passion; it's a waste of energy and you risk getting lost. Rather, you can mould your attitudes according to Taoism, tao meaning "the way", which forms both the basic principle of the Universe and the vector for its multiple transformations. Oriental philosophy is a lot more flexible than the three main monotheist religions in the way that it attempts to explain our world. It has no commandments, and neither does it forbid anything. It is also a lot more modest, since it does not deal in earth-shattering revelations or blinding flashes. Rather, it uses words and images which make you think, as would an attempt to brighten up the darkness around you by lighting a number of small candles.

When I first approached the Volunteers, I was told that there were no positions available. However, once I stated that I had a diploma in agriculture, my application was immediately accepted. After completing some preliminary placements, I was told I would be sent to Haiti. A fortnight before I was due to set off, without a word of explanation, I was told I was being despatched to Rwanda. In those days, the ex-Belgian colony had not yet become tragically notorious, and so its name meant nothing to me.

*

On 15 September 1980, after a thirteen hour flight, I landed in Kigali, along with another four volunteers who, like me, were happy but a little nervous. We were in for a two-year stretch without the slightest idea what was awaiting us. As soon as I stepped off the plane though, my senses were assaulted by the shock of a myriad of scents: the smells of earth, of dampness and of flowers all intermingled. Nature was being brought to me on the wind and was penetrating my very skin, like the perfume of a loving woman. I immediately fell under a spell.

We are soon greeted by the Volunteers' leader and by the team that we had come to relieve; they have roughly another month to serve, during which time they have to train us, in a process referred to as "tile-laying". So, I am going to learn something new. Pierre, whom I am going to replace as head of the beekeeping project, is all smiles as we step into his tarpaulin-covered 404 Peugeot, the archetypal French pick-up truck.

"We are going to pick up the post and then we'll join the others

3. HONEY FOR HOPE

for the reception at the embassy."

I am still a bit stunned, but I feel good. My whole being feels vibrant; this is my first big journey, and I am in Africa! In front of the Kigali post office, Pierre says:-

– *"Take the opportunity to look around, I'll be right back."*

Leaning our of the car window and with my eyes fixed on the horizon, I am soon enjoying a daydream when suddenly I feel something gently tapping my arm and I hear a child's voice imploring softly:-

– *"You give money"*

Everything is as I had imagined, down to the begging urchin, which is a reassuring cliché for a well-fed westerner. I turn round, about to make excuses about not having any Rwandan currency, and I receive a shock! Right beside the child there stands a leper, his face wrecked, one eye missing, no nose or ears left. His mouth is a gaping hole, seemingly bottomless and into which I feel as though I am falling, I feel nauseous. The world has just been turned upside down. Surely this cannot be; this absurd mask must be ripped off his face. Despite the heat, I shiver. Was it him or the child who touched my arm? I look at them both in turn, trying not to show my fear. In a flash I recall the scene in the film Papillon when Steve McQueen doesn't hesitate to take a drag from a cigar proffered by a leper just like this man. I try to gain reassurance by telling myself that surely if he is loose on the streets it must mean that he is not contagious. Time stands still. More beggars approach the car. One of them is suffering from elephantiasis and his lower limbs are horribly deformed. A one-legged man is hopping on crooked crutches. They are joined by a second, then a third leper. Yet amongst this assembly of cripples, I am the object of curiosity. I am the ridiculous foreigner. I am petrified and dare not move. Fortunately Pierre is coming out of the post office. Without any qualms, he sends them packing with shouts of "get the hell away from here" and sits back behind the wheel, laughing. I feel relieved that he has intervened, but also embarrassed by his brutal behaviour, which smacks of colonialism.

― *"Welcome to Africa!"*

Embarrassed, I muttered "thank you". I resent him for having played this 'new boy' trick on me, but most of all I am angry at how badly I have reacted. I have just been given a good lesson about what it is to be different.

Towards the end of the afternoon we set off for M'Bazi, a journey along dirt tracks of a mere 130 kilometres, but one which takes seven hours! When the weather is good, that is. Later it would sometimes take me up to twenty-four hours to cover the same journey!

When you are close to the equator, the sun goes down early and night falls rapidly. Darkness is complete, and of a density I am not accustomed to. We are driving through settlements of several thousand inhabitants, yet there are hardly any lights to be seen. Pierre explains that in Rwanda populations are very scattered and the notion of village as we understand it in Europe doesn't exist here. You therefore get the strange feeling that you are permanently in the middle of nowhere. At around eight o'clock we stop at one of those bars where men meet to drink amongst themselves; they have either urwagwa, which is beer made from bananas, or ikigage, sorghum beer. No women. Women are the ones who make the world go round at home and in the fields, whilst the men are busy either chatting or fighting. Machismo is found all over the world and dates back to ancient times. Man soon forgets that he is born of woman, and that she is the one who initiates him in the art of love.

The magic of electricity has not yet arrived to bring television and televised football matches. The meagre light from two oil lamps barely reaches our table. It takes some time to get used to the semi-darkness. Back in France, I would immediately have turned round at the sight of such a frightening place; our views are distorted. The owner is all smiles and offers his sole dish: goat kebabs, with or without pili-pili.

Pierre declines the pili-pili, so I ask what it is.

― *"It's a sort of chilli".*

I feel like being adventurous; a chap from the Med doesn't fear anything.

3. HONEY FOR HOPE

— *"With pili-pili please."*

As soon as the first mouthful passes my lips, it feels like I have just bitten into a piece of incandescent charcoal. It's a kebab made of live embers; I'm on fire! Pierre is killing himself laughing. Whilst I try to stem the fire that is raging in my throat by drinking three cans of coke one after the other, I can feel that everybody is looking at us inquisitively. For the second time today, I find that I am "the other" and I suddenly realise that I wouldn't much like to stroll into a bar in Nice if I were black.

We arrive in M'Bazi around midnight, and I sink into bed without even getting undressed. The introductions will have to wait until tomorrow morning. Four of us volunteers are staying in a lovely house up on a hill, not far from the administrative centre, which enables us to benefit from the availability of electricity. This is an exceptional advantage to have.

However, there is no running water, and I discover a new concept: walking water. A Rwandan employee brings us water supplies four times a day. This is vital work for him and it enables him to feed his whole family. He fetches water from a spring located approximately 500 metres further down, using a 25 litre jerry can. What's quite amusing is that if he stops along the way to have a chat, he balances the can on his head, even if it is full, as if there was nothing to it. 100 litres of water a day, for drinking, cooking, washing up, washing – and that's only half a bathtub! As for the washing of clothes, that is done using rainwater from a butt. Needless to say, during the dry season we don't change our clothes every day. You don't waste such precious natural resources for the sake of fashion!

The first time Pierre takes me to see "our" bees, he parks the car a good distance from the apiary, and produces full protective suits. I tell him of my surprise:-

— *"Let me tell you, I have been going into beehives since I was a nipper, and the only protection I have ever used is a veil; I am not afraid."*

I think back to when my aunt and myself would tend the hives in short sleeves, not minding a dozen or so stings as we were accustomed to receiving venom, as are beekeepers the world over. I can still recall my surprise rather than any anger when one particular sting was more painful than the other: "Oh what a beast! This one really hurts!"

Pierre doesn't care for my childhood memories.

- *"Put the suit on, I'm telling you."*

So it is trussed up like deep sea divers that we approach the apiary, albeit this is a pompous description for a line of five hives set on a metal bench under a galvanised sheet. The legs of the bench are stood in cans containing old engine oil; this is a modern-day version of the concept of a moat, and they are used to protect honeybees from ants, which are dreadful predators.

As we get to the first hive I ask Pierre to let me have the privilege of establishing a personal contact with these famous African bees as I am anxious to get to know them. With a bent forefinger I tap on the alighting board, as you would knock on a door, which is a standard way of assessing how a colony reacts. With normal bees, there is a bit of agitation and a few bees pop out to find out what is going on; with an aggressive colony or if the weather is stormy, four or five bees are going to make sure the intruder backs off; nothing too nasty. But today in less than one minute I have the whole swarm stuck on my face. Ten to twenty thousand furious bees! From this raging cloud comes an acrid smell of venom which sticks in my throat. I run to the Peugeot, following Pierre who had of course stayed well back. He grabs the smoker and we cover each other with smoke to try and get rid of the insects that are clinging to our protective suits, and we resume our desperate flight.

Having pursued us for a distance of three kilometres, and fought for half an hour, the bees start to give up and go back to their hive. We are coughing, spitting and suffocating with heat by the time we can at last take our jackets off. Once again Pierre is laughing his head off. I am taken aback, and as I wipe the sweat off my face, I question him:-

- *"What happened? I have never seen anything like it."*

3. HONEY FOR HOPE

— *"These are African honeybees, mate. I'm done with them, now it's your turn. And good luck to you!"*

My beginner's enthusiasm has just been seriously dampened. That night I share my concerns with him.

— *"Something has to be done, I can't work in such conditions."*
— *"Forget it, it can't be done."*

The chap before me went through the same process;

— *"These bees are seriously disturbed, you can't do anything with them. In any case you don't get much more than a couple of kilos of honey per hive, that's the local average."*

— *"What, with two flowering seasons? Are you kidding me?"*

I am speechless. Back in France, with only one harvest, annual production is around forty kilos per hive! And to think that we are supposed to teach young Rwandan farmers how to improve productivity from their traditional hives!

— *"Let me give you a piece of advice. Play it cool. Enjoy life. Remember that you are here for two years."*

Following his own principles, he settles down on the veranda, a whisky bottle within reach, and starts rolling a spliff.

— *"You see, the beauty of this stuff is that it grows wild here; all you have to do is pick it. No need for any intermediaries."*

Seeing that I am somewhat crestfallen, he makes me an offer which goes some way towards cheering me up.

— *"Tell you what, the two of us are going to go away together for ten days or so and meet up with people who practise beekeeping in this country. Maybe they'll be able to teach you a trick or two to help you along. And it will give me an opportunity to have a look around before I go home. You should always mix pleasure with business."*

Pierre is a generous man! Thanks to him I go on a dream journey. I see breathtaking landscapes. Rwanda is known as the country with a thousand hills, and it is a well deserved saying. It has impressive sheer drops, river fords, luxuriant vegetation – everything is both spectacular and sublime.

Beekeepers welcome us like long-lost brothers; some of them own up to fifty or a hundred hives, and they are delighted to share their passion with us. I feel moved when I meet these distant 'relatives' lost in the middle of the jungle who practise exactly the same craft as my aunt, using the same ancestral methods. I am delighted to discover that beekeeping is a well-established tradition in this wonderful country. Evenings are truly surreal. We drink until we are sated, each in turn dipping the only wooden pipe into the large hollowed out gourd that they have filled with local 'beer' for the notorious pipe smoking ceremony. The Chief prepares the pipe in a quasi-religious way, paying particular attention to the coating of saliva that he applies to it with his tongue, before passing it over to me with a big smile. This is the traditional way of showing that the pipe is not poisoned. It is then passed from mouth to mouth; what we are smoking is hemp of course. Only organic stuff will do…

Our encounter with some western monks is a little more peaceful, but no less rewarding. They are also beekeepers, and have been for several generations, so to speak. In exceptional years, their honey yield goes up to between five and ten kilos. I tell them of my disappointment as compared with European standards. They have a greedy look on their faces when they tell me the story of this monk who is supposed to have harvested one hundred and twenty kilos. It is impossible to disentangle myth from reality.

Towards the end of our trek, we set off to visit a well-known beekeeper in the north of Rwanda, at the foot of the volcanic mountains which form the border with Uganda. We spend hours going up and down hills, using tracks that to me seem more and more risky, whilst the farmers we meet here and there give us very vague directions. The journey is magnificent, but I am beginning to wonder.

3. HONEY FOR HOPE

- *"Do you know where we are or are you just pretending?"*
- *"You must trust in my innate sense of direction. I've spent two years in Africa, mate!"*

Mid afternoon, we finally come across a slightly better track, then another which is slightly wider, and so forth until we reach a real road and the tarmac gives a welcome break to both the 404's tired suspension and our own spines. Pierre is triumphant.

- *"what did I tell you?"*

I squint.

- *"What's that hut over there, with a barrier?"*
- *"It's probably the Ugandan border; we must be too far north. The soldiers will give us details."*

When we stop in front of the group of soldiers they immediately surround us, Kalashnikovs at the ready, threatening looks on their faces and I can feel Pierre's confidence evaporating.

- *"We're on the wrong side, he mutters between gritted teeth"*
- *"What?"*

These are Ugandan soldiers; therefore, logically, we must be in Uganda.

It will take us five hours of endless discussions to convince the officer in charge that we have crossed the border by mistake whilst looking for an elusive beekeeper, and that we are neither smugglers nor spies! The atmosphere is tense. Uganda has only emerged from Amin Dada's dictatorship, and power has already changed hands twice. The inevitable bribe eventually wins the day more effectively than any of our protestations. The man holding the gun always gets his way.

Once we set off, relieved to have got off so lightly, for the first time since my arrival I can at last tease Pierre.

- *"So, you were saying something about your innate sense of direction?"*

The story will of course do the rounds all over Rwanda!

His tour of duty is coming to an end. Like some other Volunteers, he has opted to make the return journey by crossing Africa from Kigali to Algier; he has just purchased on an old BMW600 motorbike left by the Germans at the end of the war. He is now pouring all his energy into preparations for this new adventure.

I find myself in sole charge of the beekeeping project, with the help of a joiner tasked with manufacturing the hives along with all the equipment required. The Volunteers' strength resides in their ability to work independently and to see projects through to completion with the minimum of materials, most often from nothing at all.

For example, some volunteers in another region had decided to help local farmers create rice paddies, and they spent two years wading in mud day after day in order to cultivate a few hectares. Their reward came when the delighted locals organised a big celebration to mark the first harvest.

Some others though got it completely wrong when they set up a "Rabbit Project", and they showed how a lack of understanding of local ways can stop a good idea in its tracks. At the beginning, the idea had been to provide the population with a source of food to supplement ibishyimbo, the national dish of beans that forms the basis of local nutrition. Being easy and cheap to produce, rabbit seemed the most obvious choice. So the Volunteers had built a large number of hutches, marked and fenced off a vast parcel of land to allow for rapid breeding, carefully selected a breed of particularly tough Australian rabbit and purchased a few pairs. In awe of such good intentions, no Rwandan had had the courage to tell them that none of the locals would ever bring themselves to eat those animals, which simply did not form part of the Rwandan culture. Therefore only local whites ended up buying the rabbits, which somewhat defeated the object.

In order to avoid making such mistakes, I have long discussions with M'Bazi beekeepers. Together we produce home-made smokers, using old tin cans and making the bellows from old tyre inner chambers collected from the local tip. They advise me to swap the traditional eucalyptus leaves for tobacco leaves, which calm bees down better. We

3. HONEY FOR HOPE

do manage to get some work done, despite receiving countless stings, but progress is slow and a far cry from the ambitious projects I had arrived with. I was still missing a key element.

After two months of groping around in the dark, I travel to Kigali for a meeting with the Volunteers' director and the French ambassador, a strange character who bears no resemblance to my preconceived idea of a career diplomat. He is more like a disillusioned adventurer who has arrived here by chance and already nostalgic at the thought that he will have to leave again. He is a very kind man who is very keen to get involved with our beekeeping project. I tell them straight off that I intend to stop everything. I do not wish to carry on under the present circumstances, pretending that I am getting some work done whilst going round in circles. It would be dishonest and presumptuous towards the very people we are supposed to help. I don't even know whether the project is viable. The only thing I do know for sure is that I need time to find a possible solution. I am going to go back to square one. Having at first taken me for a madman, the two men give way in the face of my determination. I think they have appreciated my sincerity.

*

I have returned to taking a long hard look into books, but thought without action gets you nowhere. I decide to go and observe bees in their own environment. I spend four months carrying out research, with the help of two Rwandan people. We sometimes spend several days in the heart of the forest, sleeping in hammocks, in total physical and mental harmony with nature. I don't know what I am looking for, or even whether I am going to find it, but I perceive instinctively that the bees themselves are the key to the solution.

I soon notice that their behaviour in the wild is quite different from what I had seen so far. When we approach a colony, there is no display of aggressiveness and we can even handle them using just a little smoke. This is surprising coming from wild bees, whereas back in M'Bazi we have sometimes seen a disturbed colony simply take off, abandoning the hive and its brood, which is a totally baffling behaviour for a beekeeper from the western world.

I even get to witness the amazing complicity that can exist between man and animals, something I thought could only happen in my dreams. At swarming time, that is to say when a colony splits into two, the new group of bees initially settles on a branch whilst waiting to find a permanent nesting site. One day we come across such a swarm "in transit", one of my assistants gracefully heaves himself to the top of the tree, more than twenty metres up; having managed to spot the queen amongst her thousands of worker bees, he delicately picks her up. In order to keep his hands free, he holds the queen between his lips and he waits patiently for the bees to come and settle on his body before carefully making his way down. Back on the ground, he places the queen into a traditional African hive, one they call a "basket" as it doesn't contain any frames, and the whole swarm settles calmly down with her. The "Bee-Man" had not received a single sting. This is an African miracle, and a moment of intense emotion.

Having completed our observations, we decide to head back to M'Bazi with a dozen full hives, some with swarms we have picked up in the forest, others with bees that we have bought from local farmers, so that we can continue our research. Having loaded the hives onto the 404's flatbed, we set off in the dead of night, so as to transport the bees quietly. Back in Europe this type of migratory bee transport is quite common and does not normally pose any risk.

Unfortunately, we incur some delays and by the time we are some fifteen kilometres from town, we are hit by the first rays of sunshine. Having been unsettled by all the bumps in the track, the bees are in a mad rage and they take flight in large clusters, pouring into villages as we drive through. By now the assistant who had sat at the back to look after the hives is desperately hammering on the roof of the cab to alert me to the disaster, but if I stop the car it will get even worse. So I put my foot down. In the rear-view mirror I can see people running everywhere with arms flailing. I too would run like mad once I had made an emergency stop just outside M'Bazi.

Once calm is restored, a brief assessment indicates that we must have shed around one hundred and fifty thousand bees in our wake!

The next day, we have to face the wrath of the village elders who have come as a delegation to the villa in order to complain about our thoughtlessness. I must admit that I would have preferred to face a swarm of bees, which I could have fled from without any sense of shame. Fortunately, the incident would not mar our friendship.

3. HONEY FOR HOPE

Week after week we and the bees are making some progress in mutual discovery. Counting, measuring, showing patience and being humble eventually reveal keys to unlock the mystery. This one in particular: African bees are a fifth smaller than their European cousins.

From the start of the project, nobody has taken into account this difference in size, and therefore in biotope, and the hives have been manufactured according to European measurements. This sums up the influence of colonialist attitudes upon beekeeping! Wrong standards cannot be applied. A hive is a world where every measurement is very precise, and where everything has its place and its function. If the space is too large, the bees are not able to organize their work or to defend themselves against predators; they cannot get their bearings and they become stressed.

Furthermore, in Europe we customarily manipulate hives during the hottest hours of the day; this is done in order to reduce the chance of chilling the colony, which needs to maintain the hive temperature at around 35°, and also to take advantage of the fact that forager bees will be away collecting. In Africa however, plants release nectar at the beginning and at the end of the day. Bees therefore forage at those times, and when we turn up out of sync in the middle of the afternoon, we are perceived as invaders.

On the strength of this new data, we set up two experimental apiaries, each with twenty hives that we have built to African standards.

As early as from the first flowering season, each hive yields seventeen kilos of exceptionally good honey! The best harvest in my whole life. From now on I will be nicknamed "The Great Beekeeper".

In accordance with oral African tradition, a Rwandan storyteller does me the great honour of recounting my story, which he tells during a celebration night in M'Bazi. Of course I can't understand a word he is saying, but his tale is punctuated by laughter and mirth coming from the people assembled around the large bonfire, and that is for me a wonderful reward. I must admit that I am proud to have achieved success, and I am also happy to be able to bring a small improvement to the life of these people whose everyday life I have been sharing for several months.

*

We were not treated as strangers. We were invited to weddings; newborn babies were introduced to us, and we were asked to pay our respects to the dead. Our car, the only motor vehicle in M'bazi, would be used as an ambulance whenever a sick or injured person, or a pregnant woman whose delivery wasn't going to plan, needed to be transported to Butare, the nearest town located some twelve kilometres away. This would only happen as an emergency or in desperation, since a visit to the hospital was considered as a last resort, and to be sought only if the local healer or dispensary nurse had reached the limits of their knowledge.

My disappointment is huge when, following this unexpected harvest, I ask the farmers whether the children have enjoyed eating the honey; they seem perplexed by my question and reply that the crop has been used mostly to chaptalise in their beer brewing! I instantly understand that we are still separated by a vast cultural gap.

Admittedly, there was no starvation in Rwanda, but the whole population was suffering from serious nutritional deficiencies. However, I had noticed that the families of beekeepers were generally in better shape than the average population. Whenever we were transferring a swarm into one of our new hives, children would rush to devour the brood combs as if it were cake, whilst their father would explain knowledgeably that cells full of larvae were very good for the children's health.

This was confirmation of everything I had heard throughout my teenage years and during my later studies about the properties of hive products. Only now I was no longer dealing with beliefs or theories, but with a tangible reality. Rwandan farmers had discovered nutritional supplements via empirical methods that were nonetheless totally effective.

These bright-eyed youngsters offered a strange contrast with the images I had of a large family I had met during one of my trips and whose memory was haunting me. I had seen thirteen children quietly lined up in front of the family hut, from the eldest to the youngest, increasingly frail, increasingly vulnerable, almost translucent – the terrible external signs of a mother who is drying up through multiple pregnancies and diminishing food resources as the family increases in numbers.

This is when the idea first came to me that the countries which,

3. HONEY FOR HOPE

out of a sense of propriety we call "developing" - when most of them are in fact sinking into misery, particularly in Africa – may already have natural resources that could be used to alleviate some of their suffering.

The ambassador is so taken by our initial results that he tells me he is going to ask the UN to take over from the Volunteers and sponsor the beekeeping project in order to develop it on a larger scale. Unfortunately, my humanitarian ambitions are stopped in their track in July when, struck down by hepatitis, I am confined to my bed.

Like many African countries, Rwanda is reputed to produce the hottest chillies and to harbour the best witchdoctors in the world. Some of them are said to be able to cure hepatitis in three days! This is taken seriously by OMS, to the point that they send out a team to carry out a field study on the efficacy of these plant-based treatments.

I had been privileged to meet one of those unusual witchdoctor characters at the beginning of the year. The village chief had very deferentially ushered me into a dark hut where the atmosphere was disturbing. The witchdoctor who was now staring at me instantly reminded me of the healer from my childhood. I sensed immediately that I was not looking at a simple chicken slaughterer, but at someone imbued with true powers, the bearer of age-old traditions.

In the same way as the light of those stars that reaches us after millions of years can tell us about the origin of the world, looking into his eyes I got the impression that I was able to instantly reach into time immemorial, when man had to live on his wits. I must admit that I was frightened. All Westerners, even non-believers, are heavily influenced by Christian teachings, and I was insidiously being told that I was facing the obscure dark forces that populate the Bible.

We must not let ourselves be blinded by our beliefs. As soon as I am struck by hepatitis, I ask one of our assistants to fetch from the witchdoctor the potion that will defeat the disease. When he gets back four days later, I have already been flown back to France. Given the seriousness of my case, nobody has been prepared to take any risks. I will never know whether the legend was true.

4. African Magic

I get back to Africa in 1985 when I find myself in Conakry, the capital of Guinea. During the previous year, Sékou Touré has disappeared and his successor, Colonel Lansana Conté, reopens his country's borders to the outside world. After twenty-six years of an implacable dictatorship, the economy is in dire straights. Since they are settled in an area bordering Côte d'Ivoire, a thousand kilometres from the capital, local coffee and cacao growers have got into the habit of selling their crops directly to France, which pays them in CFA Francs (*) rather than risk sending it to Conakry which is crippled by waste and corruption, and where you can whistle for your payment.

One of my friends has been tasked by the new government with restarting commerce for those two commodities. Knowing that I am experienced and that I love Africa, he asks me to take charge of the project. It is a matter of visiting small producers to convince them to start sending their crops to Conakry again, in order to kick-start activity in factories and the harbour there. After so many years, this is a difficult challenge, but I am attracted by the human aspect of the enterprise.

I am to fly to N'Zérékoré, which is the main town of the forested area with one hundred thousand inhabitants, aboard an old ramshackle Fokker which connects once a week, following a timetable that is never set in advance. All you have to do is turn up at Conakry airport for seven in the morning on a Wednesday, and await the airline's goodwill. That day I get lucky and we set off at twelve and the pilot, who is obviously flying this route for the first time, only goes round in circles

---

* *CFA stands for Coopération financière en Afrique centrale ("Financial Cooperation in Central Africa.")*

for half an hour before finding the unmarked runway.

My local contact is called Mamadou and he will be our wholesaler. He is a well-known trader and I soon set off with him to go round the villages. We have to gain the tribal chiefs' confidence so that they will give permission for the growers to sell their crops to us. In some places, children come forward and touch me inquisitively. They have never seen a white man! In the fields, I check the coffee and cacao plants and I inspect the beans, wearing a straw hat exactly like the chap in coffee adverts back in France!

As everywhere else in the world, it is at mealtimes that you really establish contact. We always get served the traditional dish: white rice on which is poured a ladleful of green sauce, made from pounded potato leaves or cassava leaves, smoked fish, palm oil and chillies. This is the most difficult 'test' of the day!

In N'Zérékoré, I am staying with Dr Papus, the local doctor, who has welcomed me with open arms. One afternoon as I see him donning shorts and a T-shirt, I ask:-

– *"Do you practise a sport? I'm going to football training; do you want to come along?"*
– *"Sure. I haven't played for a long time."*

After a ten minute walk, we get to the town stadium, a sad concrete construction leftover from the Marxist era, and that's when I realise only too late that Papus plays for the first team. As everyone is getting changed on the sidelines, I try to slip away, but the players are delighted to have a surprise guest.

– *"Which position do you usually play?"*
– *"Goalkeeper, but I only play as an amateur…"*

Never mind. They hand me a kit and push me ahead. During the warm up, I see the stadium is filling up with more and more people. I soon realise that my presence is the cause of this keen interest. The laughing spectators point to me. A white man in goal in N'Zérékoré! But they are not mocking me; rather I perceive an immense wave of friendship which gives me an intensely warm feeling.

4. AFRICAN MAGIC

During the match the atmosphere is delirious. Every time I stop a ball, the stadium erupts. You'd think you were in the middle of the World Cup!

I discharge my duties honourably and the match concludes with a two-two draw. However, I have just lived through a unique moment of pure happiness, by experiencing brotherhood. Word of my "exploits" soon makes the rounds. From that day onwards, I am treated as one of them, no question. All the growers now agree to sell their crops to me. The first part of my mission has been accomplished.

*

On the day of my departure, there are several of us passengers waiting on the runway below the plane, whilst the cargo is being loaded: mostly goats, chickens and bananas. The captain arrives and greets us. He is holding a red and white stick. I hardly get time to wonder about the use of such a strange accessory before he goes towards the door and attempts to insert the stick upright into the belly of the plane, which proves impossible.

– *"Too heavy. Unload the bananas!"*

I hardly dare understand that this miserable piece of wood is what he uses as his yard-stick to evaluate the weight of the plane; hasn't he got anything more precise? Once a few bunches of bananas have been unloaded, the stick goes through. I am dying to point out to the captain that his measuring does not take into account the weight of the passengers, but I fear ridicule. After all, he must know what he is doing, otherwise he would have died ages ago. You take your reassurance where you can find it.

As the aircraft launches itself in the heart-rending noise of its screaming old engines, I have the distinct impression that the undercarriage is going to get stuck in the top of the trees that line the runway. At the back of the cabin, the goats are bleating for all they are worth. As if we were in Noah's Ark, we leave the ground. I close my eyes for a few seconds. We've cleared the trees.

Back in Conakry, I have to oversee the reopening of the factory. The first few tests are both satisfying – the coffee has been well selected – and worrying: for every ten sacks of raw coffee going through the entrance, only four sacks leave through the back door. I know farmers always tend to place a few rocks at the bottom of sacks, that's part and parcel, but the ratio seems unduly high.

I therefore decide to follow the progress of the precious pods through the whole factory, and when I crawl under one of the machines I find the answer to the riddle. On the belt, the workers have installed a small plank of wood that enables them to divert some of the coffee. The grains fall directly into an underground recess, where two of them are squatting on their heels, busy filling up sacks. I am both furious and amused. "Resourcefulness" has formed part of their daily universe for so long, how can one resent their trying to find means to survive at any cost? Nevertheless, so as to gain respect, I threaten to dismiss them all on the spot. Otherwise they will treat me as a mug whom they could fleece at any opportunity.

A few weeks later, Mamadou joins me in Conakry. He has already gathered up two hundred tons of coffee. For our part, we already have our first European customer: a trading firm in Hamburg. As soon as the international money transfer is received, I call at the bank to make the biggest cash withdrawal in my life: the equivalent of seven hundred thousand French Francs. In small denominations, as we need to pay each individual grower separately.

Mamadou and I park the pick-up truck in front of the bank, and stride into the branch with guns in our belts. We each in turn load up eight enormous hessian sacks full of bank notes onto the vehicle's platform, which is being watched by a third man. We cover it with a tarpaulin and then a net which is anchored firmly to the sides. Our companion sits on top of the precious cargo, shotgun in hand, and we set off for N'Zérékoré, This is a one thousand kilometre journey over three days, only stopping for essentials like petrol or food, taking turns to sleep so as never to leave our precious booty.

When we get to our destination, after paying everybody, we load the cargo onto ten lorries and set off on the return journey. Another astounding five day journey, during which we barely get any sleep at all. Such a cargo sparks off a lot of interest, and we have to watch

4. AFRICAN MAGIC

everybody, in particular the military personnel in charge of protecting our convoy! I have learnt by experience that in this country anything can disappear without trace in an instant. And this has nothing to do with black magic. I get a feeling of being a performer in a film somewhere between "The Wages of Fear" and "Greed in the Sun"; though I have to admit that it is a thrilling feeling.

Back in Conakry, having sorted through the beans, we end up with roughly one hundred and eighty tons of pure coffee, which we immediately ship to Hamburg by boat. Standing on the jetty, I feel quite emotional as I witness the departure of our first crop…

A month later, the sky falls on my head. The Germans are cancelling their order, they demand that we reimburse the money they have already sent, and they are taking us to court! It takes me a few days to understand the reasons for their anger and establish what has occurred.

As the containers were being loaded, I have, as is customary, placed in each a small canister of a compound designed to stop any parasites breeding during the crossing. What I didn't know was that Mamadou, thinking he was doing the right thing, had gone round after me and placed a whole stack of canisters in each container! The two customs officials who were opening the containers have been intoxicated by the gas and taken to hospital. The coffee has had to be aired for several days then sold off for half its initial value. Despite these unpromising beginnings, we will carry on working with Mamadou, who discharges his duties remarkably well.

*

After two years, I hang up my coffee-buyer's apron. I am not a born dealer, and I don't feel comfortable buying at low price a product that is worth its weight in gold on western markets. We are far removed from the concept of fair-trading. What's more, growers are now being approached by men from big companies, who make them fabulous promises – which incidentally are never kept - in order to win markets. This is not a jungle I am well suited to.

I therefore go back to France, where I realise that I have lost sight of my "life path". I still have deep inside me the feeling that my quest is not over yet. I must reach the end of what I am on earth for. And first of all I have to know more about the natural medicine that I have been brushing against for so long now.

For five years I am going to seriously study Chinese medicine and acupuncture with an exceptional master, Gérard Saminadin, a doctor of Indo-Asian origin. During this training, I also touch on natural medicine, based on plants. This "green medicine" concept takes me back to the idea I had glimpsed ten years previously, and it enables me to go into more depth with my thinking on alternative solutions applicable for poor countries.

I have retained many contacts in Rwanda, and I talk about my suggestions to one of my friends, who has become Minister for Health. In November 1990, he invites me to travel to his country to explore the possibilities offered by this type of medicine, which fits in well with their traditions. The first meetings I have with the Managing Director of the Kigali hospital are very constructive. The project is on the right tracks. At least, that's what I believe.

I take the opportunity to visit neighbouring Burundi, as I have been told there is a very talented witch-doctor practising there, and that his reputation has crossed the border, which is very rare. What is even rarer is that the witch-doctor in question is a woman. But the word is too pejorative in its feminine form so rather they talk about a she-druid.

As soon as I had been told that she is capable of curing hepatitis in a few days I knew I had to go and seek her. The coincidence was too great to be simply fortuitous.

As I reach her village, her name is being uttered in a low voice, and I am taken to her hut very slowly, as though the journey itself is part of the ceremony. As I step into the darkened room, I recognize an atmosphere which is familiar to me despite the passage of time. The difference is that I am no longer scared. My mind has been opened up. The woman who welcomes me with great kindness must be in her fifties, but she doesn't look like the other African women of that age. In her eyes I can see only light and goodness. I can imagine the force of personality that she has had to exert in order to both declare and use her gifts in such a traditional and male chauvinistic African

4. AFRICAN MAGIC

community. Through her, I perceive the courage of those women in Europe who would risk being burnt alive rather than renounce their mission. This is the everlasting struggle women face to overthrow the racist barriers that have been erected in their path by men jealous of their prerogatives. The she-druid is happy to tell me about her practices. She insists on the importance of spending time listening to those who come to see her, because she is convinced, without ever having studied psychology, that part of one's suffering can be alleviated through talk.

Then she takes my hand, closes her eyes and "listens" to the energy flowing from my being and vibrating through her own body. She tells me about the multitude of plants that she uses, and of the vital importance that either moon rays or sun rays can have on them. Each treatment is accompanied by a specific diet, since illnesses always result from an imbalance in harmony between components which are all, even the tiniest one, of importance.

Day and night, yin and yang: she is not using the same words, but from thousands of kilometres away her reasoning is more or less the same as that of Chinese practitioners. Only Westerners have forgotten that man's unity rests on duality, whereas science itself has demonstrated this fully. It is a double helix in our DNA that makes up our chromosomes, which in turn are assembled in pairs. And whatever we do, the duality of masculine and feminine forms the indispensable basis of life.

At the end of our conversation, which has lasted several hours, she hands me a number of plants which symbolize the therapeutic principle, saying simply:-

– *"I know that you will carry the message, and that it will go far on its way."*

Through this gesture, I know that she considers me as one of theirs. I am deeply touched and proud to be granted a privilege that I perceive as a great mark of confidence.

I am immediately convinced that her turn of phrase applies to the current project in Rwanda. Unfortunately, a few months later the government is overthrown, bringing the experiment to a premature end. Internecine conflicts will not cease growing until the horrors of 1994.

Not so long ago, it was said that God used to come to this wonderful county every evening to rest. One night, He fell asleep too deeply, and the whole world has fallen asleep with Him.

*

Upon getting back from Rwanda, I get married and happily we soon have a baby. I am happy, but I cannot get rid of my attraction towards Africa. I feel the continent still has things to teach me.

A couple of friends, who are managing a hotel in Sierra Leone, suggest I join them. I set up home with my wife and daughter in a ramshackle house on a dream beach. Granted, we have to fetch water from a well, and we get our light from petrol lamps, but this is a good approximation of my idea of paradise. I earn a living by taking tourists out to discover local beauty spots aboard a six-seater boat. We sail as far as the Turtle Islands, of which there are nine. Seven are inhabited, and we stop off on one of them to purchase lobsters from local fishermen which we go and savour on another island, this one totally deserted. My passengers are delighted at the end of this dream-like day.

What they don't know is that the last island, named Hong, is the site of a practice that everyone thinks has disappeared: man-eating. Women are barred from the place, which harbours obscure rites as old as time itself. Young men get initiated and incantations are addressed to the "devil", the spirit of Evil which is represented with the face of a woman!

I have had the dubious privilege of landing on Hong, accompanied as I was by one of the tribal chiefs who has been introduced to me as a grand master of ceremonies. When he opened his mouth I shuddered from head to foot: all his teeth had been cut to a point, as a symbol for great man-eaters. This malaise, close to nausea, stayed with me during the whole of my visit in the company of this guide and his terrifying smile. It was broad daylight, and all I saw were special places dedicated to rituals and sacred stones. But despite the heat, my hands were frozen. The smell of death was floating all over this baleful island, which I couldn't wait to leave.

Africa is a world populated with a large number of secret societies whose rules govern life in an invisible yet implacable way, similar to what happens in the West with Masons or Opus Dei, and nothing can

4. AFRICAN MAGIC

be achieved without their influence being taken into account. I had just witnessed the most extreme side of this.

The business soon grows, thanks to a Belgian friend of mine, Luc Humbel, who also loves Sierra Leone and wants a slice of the action. However in 1992 the country is rocked by one of those coups that punctuate the African continent like so many convulsions, of which one never knows whether they announce an oncoming death or an oft-delayed recovery. We do not want to give up on our dream, and we await a return to calm, but no sooner is the new power in place that it is in turn challenged by a rebellion which breaks out in the East. Chaos sets in and tensions escalate. One night, which I will never forget, rebel soldiers burst into the house, stick their guns against our temples and loot whatever they fancy. We will end up fleeing aboard our boats, toward Gambia whose minister for tourism has stated that he was ready to welcome us with open arms.

*

Gambia is a strange country, a narrow strip of land on the banks of the river which has given it its name. At the mouth of the river, a maze of sea inlets surround islands covered in gigantic mangroves. The Saloum delta forms part of the Senegalese territory, but thanks to an agreement between the two countries we are allowed to navigate there. It is during a recce for future excursions that I hear of the existence of a female Marabout – the only one on the whole of the west African coast I am told. She claims that twenty-five years previously she has had a vision of an envoy from Mohamed, who has asked her to build a mosque on one of the islands.

She has taken her little boy with her, settled down in this inhospitable place without any drinking water, and she has got down to the task, stone by stone. Against all odds, she has achieved her task, and nowadays people come from all over the area to pray in her mosque.

When I discover the little building, of about twenty-five square metres and covered by a delicate straw roof, I am reminded of the miserable little chapel that Foucauld's father had built at the heart of the Algerian desert. I am pleased to note that the wills of God and Allah are sometimes the same.

Like the one in Burundi, the woman who welcomes me is all

sweetness and light. She takes my head in her hands, in a gesture of blessing, and I experience a marvellous feeling of well-being. We are in total communion. We slowly walk into the mosque. In the centre of this bare space it is as if the heavens are open. The faith that pervades the very walls makes it an exceptional place of prayer. I feel the same emotion as the one that reigns in the big blue mosque in Istanbul, in front of the grotto in Patmos, or under the perfect arches of the cathedral in Vézelay.

*

These two women are role models. They have managed to make their mark in a world where men have made themselves into gods since time immemorial. They have proved that healing, knowledge and spiritual teaching are not areas that men can forever keep for themselves in order to maintain women in a state of ignorance and submission. These women light up the path that their daughters will have to follow if they are to become liberated. Even though it is still a very long path.

In 1994, the nightmare returns. The military overthrow president Dawd Jawara. The army descends into the streets. We are crawling around the house while AK47 and mortar fire whistles past our ears. Tourists get evacuated. Africa has once again fallen victim to one of those perennial demons which deny her progress. In November we return to Europe.

I get the feeling that a page has been permanently turned, and I am a little lost. I find it hard to admit failure after all my years of efforts, and fabulous encounters.

Our marriage did not survive these trying times, and I settle in Belgium.

*

Three months later, I return to the Gambia with Luc. We intend to find out what is left of our boats and what we might be able to repair, but we are not very optimistic. Predictably, our discussions with the military get us nowhere.

Before we head back though, Luc persuades me to travel to Ginak, a place we have often heard about, but which we have never made time to visit. This village is situated two hours away by boat, on the other

4. AFRICAN MAGIC

side of the Senegalese border which snakes around the mangrove. As soon as we get there, Luc asks me in a detached tone:-

– *"Do you know that this place harbours a protective animal that the inhabitants are said to have venerated for thousands of years?"*
– *"No, what sort of animal is that?"*
– *"Honeybees."*

His answer hits me in the chest like a fist. After the usual palaver, during which I am dying to get going, the villagers start to dance and sing, and take us to the edge of the forest, where they stop at a respectful distance from an enormous baobab. I immediately recognize the humming that I was brought up with, and I silently walk up to the Saloum sacred bees. Some come and buzz around me. I kneel down with tears in my eyes. I had lost them, but they have found me again. They are showing me the way, I must follow them, it has always been my destiny. How could I have forgotten it?

As soon as I get back to Belgium, I get busy re-establishing the link that used to tie me to the honeybees. I read avidly, and I begin to tend a few hives in order to establish the necessary physical contact. However, all the detours I have made have not been in vain because they have enabled me to understand that honeybees could take me much farther than I had imagined.

5. The Invisible Medicine

By studying Chinese medicine, I have re-acquainted myself with many elements that I had learnt with my kung-fu master, and I have started to understand some of the phenomena which had puzzled me as a child.

This philosophy – since that is what it is – is based on the body-soul-spirit trilogy, which can be described with this simple image: the body is a piano, whose soul is the pianist, and music is the spirit born of their union. If the first two elements are not in harmony, the melody will always be discordant. The instrument and the musician cannot exist without one another. Since its origin Chinese medicine has sought to preserve this precarious equilibrium, whereas western medicine merely keeps the piano tuned up, giving technique the upper hand.

It is amusing to note that, in traditional Chinese medicine, the emphasis is placed first and foremost on prevention rather than cure. The role of a doctor is to keep his patient in good health. If the patient becomes ill, the doctor has failed in his mission.

Any disruption in the body-soul-spirit harmony opens the way to sickness. The pathology will vary according to the individual's genetic makeup and/or his or her behavioural dynamics, and the weakest organs will be attacked first. Sickness is generally a distress signal emitted by the body. It is the body's only means of expressing its malaise. Until harmony is restored, healing cannot take place, and the stress we suffer from the multiple attacks in our everyday life, which weakens our defences enormously, is one of our worst enemies. The immune system can only wage war if the spirit is at peace. In a way, it can be said that happiness is the best defence against illness.

This notion of "entirety" is an essential one. Having for a long time considered man as a giant jigsaw puzzle, with each piece allocated to a specialist who guards it jealously, our practitioners are only just beginning to take this notion into account. They are at last conceding the importance of the mind, both for the onset of illness and for its cure. Today everybody understands what a psychosomatic reaction is, which means huge progress has been made. However, oriental medicine, since the Japanese are masters as much as the Chinese are – goes a lot further. In addition to the circulations of blood and oxygen, which are essential fluids, another, invisible element has always been added: the circulation of energy.

A German professor of physics, Fritz-Albert Popp, demonstrated in 1993 that there exists a circulation system for light within our body, which corroborates the link between modern biology, traditional medicine and spirituality.

From the start, the difference has been that in the West we always concentrated on an exact anatomical knowledge extracted from the painstaking dissection of dead bodies, whereas in the East they were observing living beings. This is why they drew very different conclusions.

The meridians through which energy circulates resemble the nervous system, albeit they cannot be "seen"; not under our scientific model at any rate. However, they form the basis of acupuncture, among others.

It goes without saying that the medical profession rejects the concept of energy. Yet, where would Provence, and most of the countries around the Mediterranean, be without it? How did water diviners of days gone by manage to find water a few metres underground, using a simple hazel stick held between their fingers?

When he was teaching me acupuncture, my Chinese medicine teacher first described to me the technique, ie the 'geography' of it. But he also told me to go beyond it in order to let myself be guided by the energy that emanates from the point to be pricked, in the same way as the dowser used to let himself be "called" by water.

I do not reject classical medicine, which has enabled the human race to make enormous progress. But it has got bogged down with an absurd sense of logic which dictated that bacteria had to be destroyed at any cost. The human body was treated merely as a battlefield on which to test weapons that were becoming more and more sophisticated, and more and more powerful – without any consideration of

5. THE INVISIBLE MEDICINE

the damage done to the terrain.

The problem is, total victory is impossible, because bacteria never give up. A bacterium is a complex being, with two sides to it, as it can both be the source of life itself or kill it; the way it keeps evolving has ensured its survival since the dawn of time. Thus in 1992 only ten per cent of staphylococcus aureus bacteria were still responsive to penicillin, as against all of them thirty years previously. Today there is talk of a return of tuberculosis and other diseases that were supposed to have been eradicated.

Hospitals, the very places where we were supposed to be safe, have become synonymous with high risk due to the many antibiotic-resistant bacteria that thrive there; nowadays hospital-acquired infections contracted in hospitals are a lot more dangerous than most surgical procedures.

For its part, the pharmaceutical industry has mostly minimized what it discreetly terms "side effects" of its medicines. As with economics, growth at any cost has been favoured and this has caused terrible damage to the ecosystem that is the human body.

This is a classic example of a school of thought that only takes into account the visible part of a phenomenon, without any consideration for the chain of diabolical consequences. It is the same short-sighted behaviour that leads us to consume more and more so that one day we will end up choking on our own waste. We absurdly follow the short-term "here and now" whereas all our actions, be they individual or collective, should answer the essential question: what would happen if instead we strived for "everywhere and always"?

*

Chemical medicine is useful. It is even indispensable in some cases. However, its use must be limited, and delayed as much as is possible. It must remain the ultimate weapon. Taking the paradox to its conclusion, I would go as far as to say that it must become a form of complementary medicine, and one we turn to for extreme cases; that is to say, the exact opposite of what is happening at the moment. This discourse will take time to become prevalent, but I am certain that it will be heard eventually.

The whole history of humanity is made up of phenomena that man has known about intuitively prior to being able to demonstrate them. Energy is made up of vibrations that we feel, in a manner palpable yet not concrete, without being able to give a rational explanation.

For instance, there are places where we feel immediately at peace, and others where we feel awed or repulsed. It is their history, recent or ancient, their influence which addresses our senses directly.

Lamartine formulated the question: "Inanimate objects, do you possess a soul?" and I would not hesitate to answer "yes". We do not feel the same emotion when standing in front of a piece of furniture produced by a machine churning out thousands of identical objects as when looking at a piece that a master craftsman has manufactured by hand. When it comes to human beings, it is even clearer: there are people we immediately feel "in tune" with (to pursue the musical metaphor) before having even exchanged any words with them. Not to mention the alchemy that is sexual attraction, something even more mysterious, although we do now know that hormones have a role to play!

There is an endless palette of diverse sensations in respect of man's "other dimensions". For instance, the strange conviction that you are living a situation for the second time in every identical detail, or the feeling of having been someone else, somewhere else, in the past. And what about all those people who have experienced their own deaths, floating above bodies that their souls had departed?

To describe such phenomena, we often talk about a sixth sense, with no need to add anything. I would rather say that it is an intense, wider, more conscious use of the senses that we already possess and which enables us to appraise everything. Some people, be it spontaneously or due to disability, have discovered to what extent they could push the exploration of those extraordinary tools, whereas the majority of us under-estimate their power, simply because we have not learnt to develop our brain's fantastic potential.

We are talking about a musician with "perfect pitch", who can identify a note to the eighth tone, but also about Joan of Arc, or Mother Teresa, "hearing" mysterious voices that propel them towards an extraordinary destiny. We are talking about the nose of a wine expert or a perfumer, who are able to distinguish within a single scent

5. THE INVISIBLE MEDICINE

the countless nuances of fruit, flower or earth. We are talking about a painter or a photographer who knows how to "see" another reality, who looks through it and behind it. We are talking about the power of Proust's famous Madeleine. And we are of course talking about the beekeeper who knows, from the slightest whir in the hive, what the bees want him to know.

If we give them time and opportunities, our senses open the door for us to all that is universal, of the moment and forever.

Some men are capable of stroking adders; some can let tarantulas run along their arms. Others calmly swim among sharks, and Dian Fossey used to "talk" with gorillas in the Rwandan mountains. They all confirm that old beliefs, which are at the root of fear and withdrawal, are our worst enemies. Modern man finds it difficult to open up towards others and towards the unknown. This, however, is the only way he can find his true place in the world, not by standing outside of nature, or above it, but by being a simple link in the chain of life.

It was a terrible shock when we discovered that we are not at the centre of the universe, the way we had always been led to believe, and that the only thing that revolves around us is the moon. It has taken the Church five hundred years before Galileo was rehabilitated, and his message still hasn't got through. In order to compensate for his disappointment, man has imagined, and still believes, that he is at the centre of the earth. He has tirelessly tried to forcibly domesticate nature. But by violating nature, not only is he not begetting any children, he is destroying his own children's future. Saint-Exupery said it better than anyone: "We do not inherit the earth from our parents; we borrow it from our children."

6. Apitherapy

The sanitary situation of our planet is similar to its status in matters of food: totally incoherent, and scandalous. Whilst the inhabitants of rich countries are succumbing to an overdose of useless but lucrative pills, those in poor countries cannot even get their children vaccinated against diseases that western medicine can easily control. To add to the paradox, western medicine is a luxury these poor cannot afford, whilst all around them there are plants and bees that are would-be benefactors ready to oblige. However, research is in the grip of a few large laboratories where the only thought is of commercial and financial gain. The people in the labs know nothing about the human being who should be at the forefront of their concern. The only way we will be able to stop this infernal arms race that is the pursuit of profits for shareholders will be through 'green' medicine.

I suddenly see my experiences in Rwanda in 1980 and 1990 in a new light. This has to be my starting point, incorporating all the scientific and cultural elements that I have garnered in the intervening years. Products from the hive will form the basis for a new form of therapy, but they will not constrain it. This is how aroma-honeys are born.

It is simply a case of mixing honeys, in specific proportions, with essential oils from certain aromatic plants; essential oils are the active extracts obtained by distillation. The result will be a range of "cocktails" whose efficacy will be equal if not superior to that of chemical remedies. This new "apipharmacopoeia" if I dare coin a new term, will be free of negative side effects, in my view the most important element, and will offer enormous economical advantages – something very precious for people whose life is so cheap.

At the end of 1994, I talk about this concept to one of my friends, a GP in Limoges, and he tells me that a renowned surgeon, Professor

Bernard Descottes, head of department at the town's teaching hospital, has for several years been conducting trials using honey for wound healing on his patients. We are not talking about small cuts and grazes here, but about severe wounds resulting from either major surgery or serious accidents. Knowing how reticent medical 'big wigs' usually are about this type of treatment, I figure this doctor must be exceptional. A practitioner who transgresses the rules established by the scientific community runs the risk of being seen as a heretic in the eyes of those supercilious guardians of the dogma who sit on the General Medical Council, and who are as ready to use the tool of excommunication as they are a scalpel. I immediately set off for Limoges to meet him.

Sure enough, from the onset we are on the same wavelength. This man is direct and warm. He outlines the remarkable work that his nursing team has achieved and he explains that his research has been ongoing for some ten years. Part of the way has been cleared, but he still has to surmount a few obstacles. To my great surprise, he offers me a chance to help in his research. I am naturally delighted to accept. There are already a large number of scientific publications on the health benefits of honey, resulting from hundreds of pieces of work, but this clinical project is the first of its kind in France.

Our collaboration will last for two years. Professor Descottes gives me more or less carte blanche to set up tests which will complement the clinical trials in order to obtain results that will be valid in the eyes of the scientific community. At the beginning, I naturally have to fight prejudices in certain wards where people find it difficult to accept the presence of someone who is an 'outsider' in more senses than one. Not only am I from outside the teaching hospital, but what's more I am not from a medical background. Therefore I do not really have any status, which in such an extremely partitioned and hierarchical society is seen as an unacceptable drawback. As a result, the first few meetings I chair on my own are a little fraught. People from the different hospital services ask me in what capacity I propose to give directives. Their general opposition is divided equally between open hostility and passive resistance.

For his part, Professor Descottes has to face barely concealed warnings from his peers in relation to the risks he is taking by opting for the "road less travelled". Being a determined man, he soon informs

6. APITHERAPY

them that, from Hippocrates to Avicenna, honey has always been part of the great ancient healers' pharmacopeia, and that his experiments are fully aligned with the most orthodox of traditions.

However, the ambient mistrust forces him to work in somewhat peculiar conditions. Since the honey he is using cannot be purchased by the hospital pharmacy as it has not been validated by the bacteriology team, it needs to be procured through the catering department, as though it were a food supplement!

I will have to exert high levels of diplomacy to convince everyone, step by step, of the validity of my undertaking. I spend hours presenting arguments, drawing on my scientific background, but also speaking of my anecdotes from Africa and bringing in aroma-honeys to treat minor ailments: sore throats and chronic sinusitis, which the chemical-based medicine they believe in so strongly has not managed to defeat. By force of patience and determination, the magic eventually starts to work. Which just goes to prove that scientifically-minded people are receptive to the idea of experimenting on themselves! Once I have overcome these little human difficulties, we begin to work in a better environment and our common efforts soon give rise to a remarkable pharmaceutical theory on the antibacterial properties of honey.

We are able to demonstrate the total efficacy of honeys and aroma-honeys against fourteen different strains of bacteria, chosen from the most widespread within hospitals and including some strains which have become resistant to traditional antibiotics.

Obviously, products for medical use must be of a vastly superior quality to those consumed traditionally in terms of bacterial contents. In order for honey to be accepted by the hospital pharmacy, and for its therapeutic qualities to be exploited, it must arrive in a state of near-perfect purity, as it exists in the honeycomb, before it can be contaminated by man.

We therefore set up a standardization chart that imposes draconian hygiene rules upon the beekeepers who supply us. Whereas the first batches of honey we look at contained six hundred CFUs (colony forming units) per gram, we reduce this level, which is used to measure the bacterial or other micro-organism contents, down to thirty – all thanks to the new procedures followed by beekeepers during harvesting and packing. In particular, and this is something unusual for honey producers, the honey is to be packed in small 50 gram pots, in order to limit the risk of contamination during various manipulations. It is the first time that such strict standards have been put in place in the world of apiculture.

When it comes to applying the honey to a wound, Professor Descottes's team have perfected a technique that consists in cleaning wounds by brushing. Then the honey is carefully spread onto the area, and covered with gauze. During the first few days, honey has a powerful cleansing effect which can be seen with the naked eye in the form of a very dirty dressing and a very clean wound. Thereafter, a nourishing effect can be observed, which leads to very good healing. For infected wounds, thyme honey and lavender honey have exceptional healing properties. We also use honey/essential oil mixtures, which work marvellously well on difficult cases.

I remember helping a couple in Brussels with a thirteen months' old little girl who had been scalded by a pan of boiling milk, and whose arm had third-degree burns. Thanks to our procedure, I was able to avoid her having to undergo the trauma of an operation under general anaesthetic, which would have been necessary in order to undertake a skin graft; instead, within three weeks we obtained a perfect cicatrisation, which left hardly any scarring.

News of the success achieved by the "Descottes Team" soon spreads beyond his department and more and more patients are referred to him; they suffer from dreadfully infected wounds that have until then resisted traditional treatments. He obtains spectacular results. Such a gentle method, which you would expect would be slow to have any effect, turns out to be thirty to fifty percent faster-acting than chemical methods.

From a more down to earth perspective – it is well known that the cost of medicine is of great importance – our therapy presents indisputable advantages. First of all, the speed of healing means a reduction in the length of hospital stays, hence a reduction in costs. Secondly, our pot of honey is invoiced at one hundred to one hundred and twenty Francs per kilo, whereas the price of the wound-healing product which is normally used after surgery is three thousand Francs per kilo! There again, for me what really matters is the pleasure I derive from seeing a patient who suffers significantly less and who

6. APITHERAPY

is made more comfortable by the use of a treatment free of the side effects inherent to traditional chemical treatments, whilst being able to go home sooner. I must admit that I am also very proud to see, at last, the humble honeybee reinstated to the important role it deserves within a civilisation that has all but forgotten its roots and its traditions.

*

We are not alone in this fight. In Cremona, Italy, a renowned surgeon, Dr Franco Feraboli, is also performing "miracles" in his trauma department, thanks to propolis. This is a resinous substance that honeybees harvest from tree buds and bark; it is used within the hive as both the perfect insulation material and a perfect antiseptic. Dr Feraboli injects propolis straight into the heart of purulent wounds that carry streptococcus or staphylococcus that have hitherto resisted all known antibiotics, and he manages to save patients' limbs, which had otherwise been predicted to require amputation or, in the worse scenario, cause deadly septicaemia.

I meet this amazing man at an apitherapy congress on the banks of Lake Como and he informs me that, despite undeniable results, he has to carry out his work in secret so as not to attract the attention and ire of "official" medical bodies. As was the case in the Middle Ages, the "Inquisition" is keeping watch!

After getting back to Europe, I have renewed my contacts with the world of beekeeping through the organization that federates the world's apiculturists and represents six million members: Apimondia. The man now in charge, Raymond Borneck, used to be vice-president in 1980 during my first stay in Rwanda; he had visited us after our "miraculous" crop, and I therefore find myself in well-known territory.

In the Spring of 1995 whilst reading a professional publication, I come across a report about Dr Theodore Cherbuliez, president of the American Apitherapy Society, and I instinctively know that I must contact this exceptional man. His New York telephone number is at the bottom of the article and I have no difficulty in reaching him. He very kindly accepts my call and suggests we meet in a couple of months in Switzerland, his country of origin, which he visits on a regular basis.

Dr Cherbuliez's first profession is that of a child psychiatrist, a discipline he now teaches in New York and Geneva, and in which he has been a prominent figure for more than thirty years. His interest in bees started some twenty years ago, and he has soon progressed from 'amateur' to 'enlightened'. He had installed a dozen hives in the garden of his American home, and was tending them lovingly during his rare moments of leisure. He had been suffering from rheumatism, and he gradually noticed a decrease in discomfort after starting this new hobby. With remarkable intuition, he quickly established the link with the bee stings he was receiving on a regular basis, as do all beekeepers. He mentioned this to Charles Mraz, who has since died at the ripe old age of ninety four, and who is regarded as the father of apitherapy. Charles Mraz confirmed Dr Cherbuliez's observations. Bee venom does indeed have an anti-inflammatory effect on joints. From then on, Dr Cherbuliez became fascinated by the honeybee and its powers, and he couldn't wait to carry out in-depth studies - until he would in turn become a recognized expert.

In the United States, apitherapy is a few years ahead of Europe. Sixty thousand patients are treated each year, and the American Apitherapy Society has hundreds of members. There is a slight difference compared to Europe in that over there apitherapy is mostly focused on bee venom, and most of their work is based on its properties in the field of rheumatism and auto-immune conditions such as multiple sclerosis or Parkinson's disease.

In Geneva, Dr Cherbuliez welcomes me to his sister's apartment and we are surrounded by trinkets and touching memorabilia. He is exactly as I had imagined him: he smiles a lot, he is incredibly open and positive. He mixes together the wisdom of the experienced seventy year-old he has become with the inquisitiveness of the young man he still is deep down. Although at first he is a little surprised, he soon shows interest in the numerous possible uses of hive products that I let him glimpse. To support my claims, I have brought along a small case containing all the necessary ingredients and right in front of him I prepare an aroma-honey with digestive properties, based on thyme and rosemary, and he samples it straight away. At the first mouthful I see his eyes light up. His enthusiasm fills me with joy.

We meet again in September in Lausanne, where the Apimondia congress is being held that year. From the start, Raymond Borneck asks Dr Cherbuliez whether he would consider taking over, for a short

6. APITHERAPY

while, the Apitherapy commission, which its absentee president has left dormant. Dr Cherbuliez is willing to accept the task, and he manages it perfectly.

Sometime later, "chance" intervenes again. I receive a telephone call from Toulouse. The caller, Robert, is suffering from multiple sclerosis. He is wheelchair-bound and cannot use his limbs. He has heard about the use that Americans make of bee venom to treat this condition and he is asking me for help. I have no experience whatsoever in this field, and I am reluctant to respond, whilst at the same time feeling unable to refuse such a request.

After a long conversation with Théodore Cherbuliez I am won over. He is going to teach me the famous bee venom therapy which is currently being practised in the United States. This is a process which, initially, has people terrified since it consists in applying bee stings "directly": it is essentially an acupuncture session where the traditional needle is replaced by the bee's stinger. In concrete terms, the bee is carefully picked up between the two prongs of a large pair of tweezers, and applied on the skin at the exact location where you want it to sting. The operation is then repeated with other bees, up to fifty times if necessary. This may seem like a huge quantity of venom, but it is quite bearable since the patient's body has already been partly numbed by the disease. As the treatment progresses, one of the patient's biggest emotions resides precisely in the recovery of pain. This is what proves that the body is coming back to life.

This technique has been given a lovely name: apipuncture. If the patient is too sensitive, it is possible to remove the stinger from the bee and to apply it as you would a needle for several micro-injections. Some practitioners use capsules containing apitoxin, which is venom which has been collected and dried for storage, but there is a question mark over its efficacy. It goes without saying that various tests are carried out on the patients beforehand to ensure that they are not allergic to bee venom; however, those presenting with a real intolerance represent a tiny percentage of the population. This could be due to the fact that being stung knowingly reduces the level of stress otherwise due to fear.

*

The plan is for me to spend some time with Dr Cherbuliez so that he can train me to use apitherapy. At the same time, I will impart my knowledge of aroma-honeys. Our collaboration is bound to be beneficial for sick people.

*

Laurence was suffering from multiple sclerosis. The homeopath who was treating her had run out of therapies and the disease was progressing inexorably, depriving her of physical strength to the point where she was no longer able to cut up her own food and was reduced to using a wheelchair every time she left the house. The degradation was reaching her brain and she was being denied the simple pleasures of writing, reading or watching television.

We tell her from the start that the treatment is going to entail an initial phase which will be very difficult to bear. Indeed, the first few venom injections trigger a violent reaction which looks like an allergic reaction, whereas it is simply a progression from the chronic state of the illness to an acute process, showing that the treatment is taking effect. This concurs with the formula that I use nowadays: "Crisis precedes healing."

Laurence decides to trust us. She is a determined woman, very independent-minded, who has until recently worked as a social worker. She does not want to accept the slow decline that is affecting her, and she shows whole-hearted determination.

Having completed the preliminary tests, we start with the treatment at a dose of two stings twice a week, up to a level of twenty injections twice a week.

Laurence stoically endures two months of serious upheaval, during which time we endeavour to reassure her. She suffers faintness, high temperatures, diarrhoea, and vomiting – all very violent, but she does not relent. Despite all the outward signs of rejection, she knows that the venom is doing her good.

She is right, and her courage is rewarded. Having battled through the terrible upheavals, which would have led others to give up, she begins to feel the first positive effects of the cure.

Initially, people around her notice that her eyes are clearer. Then problems associated with incontinence begin to disappear, and her mobility and alertness improve daily, until she is once again able to

6. APITHERAPY

watch a whole film. This is an immense victory for someone whose attention span had been reduced to just a few minutes.

A year into the treatment, she is once more totally independent; she is even able to drive again, and it makes her very proud to be able to get about without assistance. It will take another two years until she fully recovers her voice, which had been severely affected.

Ten years later, Laurence will once again walk on her own two feet. She will experience the joy of seeing the birth of three grand-children and she will lead a normal life, with two weekly sessions of some fifty stings each. Her GP is lost in admiration but, paradoxically, her neurologist won't have anything to do with her anymore! As I write she has now been enjoying this new lease of life for sixteen years, thanks to the honeybee.

*

Sarah had also been struck down by multiple sclerosis. She was a very active woman, whose doctor had just recommended she use a walking stick; she couldn't bear the thought.

Like Laurence, Sarah refuses to let the disease progress without doing anything about it. She describes to us the ordeal of constant pain that all her fellow sufferers endure: the awful feeling that her body is grasped in a vice which tightens a little more every day.

Again we take the time to clearly explain the procedure and its different stages. To have a perfectly well informed patient, who subscribes totally to the treatment, is one of the keys to success. Despite being decidedly apprehensive, Sarah resolves to embark on this adventure.

The treatment immediately triggers a massive crisis, with a serious worsening of her symptoms to the point where she is bed-bound for several days. But again perseverance pays off. Six months later, Sarah puts on her running shoes and can once more enjoy her jogging.

She will later get married and move to Chicago, where Théodore Cherbuliez will refer her to a therapist known to him for further treatment. In a country free of hang-ups, the therapist is able to tell journalists about the spectacular progress "her" patient has made, which means Sarah is featured in several press articles.

Her husband having to travel frequently on business, she accompanies him and has the bees she needs for her treatment delivered by courier to the various hotels where she stays. She has told Théodore about the endless mirth that can be caused by the arrival of those packets containing hundreds of humming insects. Each time the very worried receptionist calls her to explain that he has just accepted on her behalf a box that emits a truly terrifying noise. The fear of the 'killer bee' is so widespread in that country that the poor man cannot for one moment imagine that these insects are here to save her life.

*

People who come to us have often exhausted all the resources that conventional medicine can offer once it has failed to alleviate their suffering. This is not for the want of means or knowledge. Most often, the lack of time and ability to listen is key. Each pathology is ascribed a standard treatment, and those that do not conform to the norm are condemned to being shunted from one practitioner to the other until the register of known specialist conditions is exhausted.

*

Renée had been suffering for seven years (!) with chronic infections that had resisted all the established antibiotics and cortisone treatments - those from the pharmacopeia of course. Genital herpes, skull psoriasis, multiple mouth ulcers, hospital acquired staphylococcus aureus: her immune system had been wiped out.

When she arrived, wearing a dressing-gown, accompanied by her sister-in-law who was helping her stand up, she was in a state of acute weakness and total readiness to give up.

We immediately start a course of aroma-honeys which gradually gives her some relief. But after a year, despite clear improvements, I feel we are only treating the symptoms. We have not yet found the root-cause of the problem.

We sent for an analysis of her hair, something that is quite common in the States, and the truth finally shone through: this woman had suffered mercury poisoning. Her blood contained eight times the maximum accepted dose!

We groped around a little more to identify the cause, but there was no need to dig very deep: it was talked about a lot in the media at the time; it was in the mouth.

6. APITHERAPY

From the moment her dentist started, once a month, to carefully extract her many fillings, she was on the road to a complete recovery.

*

Official medicine has invented the term "alternative" to describe all those who practise a different form of healing. It is as though the two paths were never to meet; however, when all is said and done, they complement one another.

*

Carole brought us a three-months old baby suffering from chronic constipation.

Very quickly she confessed that she was visiting us behind the back of her husband, a well-known surgeon. He was convinced that there was a physical problem and was ready to have the child operated on, whereas she wanted to explore other avenues before taking such a drastic step.

We ask her to simply give her infant a few grains of fresh pollen, in very small, eight-times-a-day doses, and we assure her that a couple of weeks should suffice to get things back to normal.

Twelve days later, the baby has gone back to having regular and normal motions.

The father immediately calls us to thank us and to invite us to dinner. This proves to be a very constructive evening, which enables us to exchange knowledge about the two "opposite" worlds to which we belong.

By a strange twist of fate, we would later be the ones sending him a patient, a nineteen-year old young lady whose life he would save.

Janice has come to see us because everyone believes she is mad. That day, Théodore is away and I see her on my own. The psychiatrist she has consulted has diagnosed severe episodes of manic depression and has started to talk about having her interned in a psychiatric hospital.

It is true that her odd looks don't do her any favours. She is dressed in neo-punk, her hair is a mess, she sports various piercings – I immediately think that she has probably been using dangerous substances. She reads my thoughts, and declares that she has never gone further than the odd 'spliff', but I find this hard to believe. I think she can't bring herself to tell me, and, until I find out more, I give her an aroma-honey designed to clean up her hepatic system, which I believe must be full of toxins.

When she comes back, accompanied by her father, he describes his "previous" daughter as a studious and happy young lady. Nothing to do with the character you think you can detect at first sight, and which is just a matter of fashion.

Théodore and I have the same brainwave at the same time. We ask whether she has undergone exploratory brain scanning to see whether she hasn't got a tumour. The stunned father replies that she has not. We recommend that he should visit our surgeon friend, and we telephone him immediately.

The examination will reveal a tumour, fortunately benign, which had probably resulted from a non-diagnosed meningitis episode. That day, Janice calls us in tears and simply says: "Thank you for listening to me when I said I was not mad."

*

Upon my return, I call Robert and he comes to Brussels with his wife. They will only stay for two months, enough time for her to learn to sting her husband on her own. The "bee venom therapy" is going to relieve him significantly and give him back a quality of life that chemical medicine, despite its powerful armoury, didn't allow. Little by little, this man is going to regain the use of one arm and he will once more be able to accomplish simple gestures.

On the day that he manages to scratch himself for the first time in such a long period, he cries with happiness. His wife phones me immediately to tell me about their very emotional moment and to thank me. Their joy overwhelms me to the very bottom of my being.

*

Bees have not ceased to astonish me. Neither have men sometimes. In the spring of 1996, I hear a great deal of praise from a friend about a book written by a well-known and well-respected Sufi master, Sheikh Bentounes:- 'Sufism, the heart of Islam'. While reading this book, I get a very intense feeling about the author's personality. My friend tells me that he has settled in the south of France, near Nice, where he heads a

6. APITHERAPY

commune, and I decide to pay him a visit next time I visit my family. Once again a simple telephone call is enough to make arrangements. The most important people are often the most available.

A month later, standing in front of the gates to the villa in which Sheikh Bentounes lives in Bar-sur-Loup, I have a moment of doubt. France has just fallen victim to another wave of Islamic terrorism attacks. What have I come to look for, exactly? But it is too late to go back now.

The person who has welcomed me takes me to a pergola where the master is sitting, surrounded by a few of his disciples. He greets me with great courtesy and asks me about my occupation, before he offers to take me round the estate. To my huge surprise, he asks whether one of his female disciples can join us. I am pleased to accept, delighted as I am that a woman is for once afforded what is considered a privilege.

My astonishment is even greater when, during our stroll, I discover a boy-scout camp under a clump of trees! Seeing my incredulity, Sheikh Bentounes smiles as he tells me that he is fighting to create a "Muslim scouting movement", because he very naturally considers that the Baden-Powell ideal of "serving others" deserves to be taught to youngsters from all countries and all religions. Obviously, the catholic hierarchy doesn't view this commitment very favourably, and his movement has already been banned in some countries, for fear it could become a hotbed of extremism. "What makes for a hotbed of extremism," he tells me, "is precisely when you don't dare to accept such things." I know I have done the right thing coming here.

Our conversation moves on to the importance of youth, its implications for the future of the planet, and of course for bees – for which we share an immense passion. He tells me about the sacred rocks of the Atlas mountains, about their initiation role in Islam, and the benefits of honey which the Koran so often recommends. I explain to him at length what my concepts are, the progress with our work so far, and, as I did with Théodore Cherbuliez, I offer to let him sample one of my aroma-honeys. He is totally seduced by the project and he pronounces a sentence that touches a deep chord within me: "This is the future."

He then makes me a magnificent offer, which takes me by surprise. To look after the setting up of a sacred apiary which he wants to establish in his commune. I am very touched and I accept immediately. Sadly, the development of my activities within Apimondia will later force me to decline his offer, to my infinite regret.

*

To limit oneself is to limit others. Fear invites hatred, which engenders violence. We need to open wide the doors and windows of our inner house, without fear of what may come in. And we must practise what we preach.

Therefore, at about the same time, I attend lectures about the Torah and the cabbala which are given in Brussels by one of the three female rabbis to officiate in the world. She lives in New York but travels regularly to her native Belgium.

I am the only man in this little group of some fifteen people, because no Jewish "male" worthy of the name can accept the teaching of a woman, and I am the only non-Jew, which does not cause me any problem because I have long since ceased to think in terms of affiliation to any specific system of belief.

Later I will speak about apitherapy with this very talented and highly educated woman, with whom I forge a deep friendship, and her enthusiastic reaction will confirm that I am on the right path. It is as if I had had to reassure myself, with her, as with Sheikh Bentounes, that honeybees always belonged to universality.

6. APITHERAPY

7. The Humanitarian Solution

In February 1997, I travel to Cuba for the first time. As soon as I step off the plane, my memory recognizes some of the bewitching scents that I once breathed in Africa. Due to jet lag, time has mercilessly slowed right down and I have lost my bearings. This is a delightful sensation.

I settle down in a small hotel at the heart of Havana's old town. I will have to wait until the following day before I can form a better idea of what I have only guessed at through the taxi's windows.

This is a town of contrasts: beauty and desolation. To start with there are the houses with their magnificent architecture which is a relic from Spanish colonisation, but time has gnawed at them little by little and they threaten to crumble and take their past with them.

There is a clash of cultures. You pass without any form of transition from Fifth Avenue to Revolution Square! A veritable armada of large US cars straight from the fifties American dream, although they stopped being imported in 1960, is still miraculously on the road, whilst puny Ladas supplied by communist "brothers" proudly square up to the monsters from enemy powers. This is a blatant symbol of the David and Goliath struggle that has been going on for so long and in which, the height of contradiction, the ubiquitous Dollar confines the Cuban Peso to small local transactions.

A friend has given me contact details for Adolfo Perez Pineiro, who is Research Director at the Beekeeping and Apitherapy Institute in Havana, and has asked me to call on him if I get the chance. Even without knowing him, I instinctively guess that I need to meet this man. I leave several messages for him during the course of my visit, but only manage to get through to him on the day before my departure. Adolfo speaks very good French, which he has learnt during his six-months stay at INRA(*) near Avignon.

As I walk into his office, I understand that I was right. Without having met before, we already 'know' each other as though we were brothers. Adolfo bears a strange resemblance to Lenin, with added kindness. Behind his round spectacles, his eyes are twinkling with mischief. Our conversation lets me glimpse fabulous prospects. As I am about to leave, I get an overwhelming idea; without even thinking it over, I offer to organize an apitherapy course in Havana.

– *"Are you serious?"*
– *"Do I look like I'm joking?"*

So we make arrangements for the following year. It is only when I am sitting on the plane that I realise the scope of my undertaking. Fortunately, Théodore Cherbuliez, to whom I relate all this as soon as I get back, is immediately taken by the idea. His knowledge, experience and total commitment will go a long way to help achieve this project, which at the moment seems to belong to the realm of utopia.

*

That Autumn, Apimondia celebrates its hundredth anniversary and, to mark the occasion, its two-yearly congress is held in Anvers, birthplace of the organization's founding member. This time, Dr Cherbuliez is elected as President of the Apitherapy Commission, and I accept his request to become vice-president.

We meet up with Adolfo, who is accompanied by some of his team. He introduces us to the Cuban Ambassador to Belgium, a very humble man to whom we give a detailed explanation on the potential of this new medicine. I think this first meeting will go a long way to obtain the necessary authorisations for the first conference.

In February 1998, Théodore and I, along with three members of the Apitherapy Commission, are welcomed to the Finlay Institute, which is the equivalent of the Pasteur Institute in Paris, and whose Director, Concepcion Campa Huergo and her team discovered one of

---

* INRA Institut National de la Recherche Agronomique, the French National Institute for Agricultural Research.

7. THE HUMANITARIAN SOLUTION

the vaccines against meningitis in 1989. This extraordinary woman, who is a member of the State Council, is a modern scientific 'brain' who has no preconceived ideas; neither has she any fears about investigating "green" medicine. In front of us is an audience of some thirty people, amongst whom are some important members of the Health and Agriculture Administrations, since bees occupy the middle ground between both groups.

Adolfo has already completed a number of projects, relating to honey of course but also on Cuban red propolis, on pollen from the royal palm, on mixtures of honey and propolis (propohoney), honey and pollen (panhoney) and honey with royal jelly; but as always, no man is a prophet in his own country, and there has been some serious fallout at clinical level.

Our more extensive experience, the new elements we bring, the more global approach we are offering, and our international status all confer upon us an advantage which immediately ensures that our speech is well received. I must admit that I am surprised at the positive response it receives. In Cuba I find an open-mindedness which is at odds with the CNN-induced image of a 'communist stronghold'. This may be due to the fact that since the revolution its inhabitants have been forced to find original solutions to problems for which they had no external help.

We have to bear in mind that, for those forty years, the illiteracy which had hitherto affected one in three people has been almost eradicated. Furthermore, Cuba prides itself in having the lowest rate of infant mortality in the world, and in being the world's largest 'exporter' of doctors. Western countries could do worse than mull over these figures, which upset received ideas about the land of cigars and salsa.

Naturally we tend to think that apitherapy, and green medicine in general, presents first and foremost an interesting solution from a financial point of view for countries in the thralls of grave economic difficulties. Just to be clear, we explain to the Cubans from the onset that we are categorically not talking about medicine at knock-down prices, but about a giant promise of progress. They are soon attracted by this paradoxical approach which consists in innovating whilst going back to basics.

*

On the other side of the Pacific ocean, Japan gives us undoubted confirmation that green medicine does not equate to poor medicine. There, remarkably, apitherapy is gradually taking place on the preventative front as well as for cures, and in-depth research is being carried out on the role it could play in the fight against cancer. The annual turnover, which is constantly rising, for propolis exported from Brazil has reached the staggering sum of 1,200,000,000 dollars, and the large Japanese pharmaceutics consortiums predict that by 2015 the turnover for green medicine will exceed that of chemical-based medicine.

In 1999, Théodore Cherbuliez and I are honoured to receive an invitation from Professor Mitsuo Matsuka, who is a member of the commission and president of the Asian Apiculture Association, to give a lecture in Tokyo under the auspices of Tamagawa University.

We talk about bee venom therapy, about standardizing products from the hive and about green medicine in front of two hundred and fifty people who are listening attentively and with passion; some have come from Australia, New Zealand and South Korea. During our stay, we also visit a clinic where a master in oriental medicine introduces us to traditional healing: the application of suction cups to prepare the body for apipuncture by means of micro-stings, and a restorative bath in warm sulphurous water. In this institution, he is the one who supervises the "standard" doctors, in what seems like a topsy-turvy world. For now at least...

*

In the face of the very keen interest sparked by our initial conference in Havana, it has been decided to set up another one, and most importantly to develop our research in a more pragmatic manner. For the first time, Cuba's isolation, which had been a weakness, is going to be a positive asset. Like everywhere else, there are undeniably some doctors who are in favour of allopathic medicine, but large laboratories do not have at their disposal a solid base upon which they could become established with the same power as in the West. Anything is still possible.

In the scientific world, no theory can be of any value until it has been confirmed using very strict protocols. However, with green

7. THE HUMANITARIAN SOLUTION

medicine, such protocols are very difficult to put into place. Since it is not possible to create a placebo that would be perfectly identical to the natural product, you cannot use the famous double-blind test technique, which consists in treating two groups of people suffering from the same disorder without either the patients or the doctors knowing who is receiving the active medicine and who is taking the placebo so that the results cannot be distorted. We therefore need to think about creating a new assessment method based on procedures. This consists of comparing the results from a series of tests against a sample group treated with conventional products. This is what is known as a randomized trial.

After several trips we are able to draft the protocols and to have them validated by the scientific ethics commissions from both the health and agriculture ministries. Like everywhere else in the world, we have to battle seemingly unavoidable administrative slowness and obstructions but little by little we manage to advance our ideas.

In February 1999, the whole of the apitherapy commission, ie about ten people, travels to Cuba for a week-long series of lectures. Théodore and I are given the title of Permanent Visiting Professors at the Calixto Garcia University of Medicine which is a nice surprise and a very moving moment in our lives.

But our most important and most anticipated reward comes when our activities receive official recognition from the faculty's Ethics Council and Scientific Council. From now on the Ministry for Health invites us to spend a week in every month on the island in order to teach, set up our scientific protocols and look after the practical applications within hospitals.

Once we have received this green light, the project takes shape rapidly. An apitherapy department, headed by Doctor Celia del Toro Hung, is opened at Calixto Garcia hospital, along with a department for applied experimentation within hospital environments. The activity soon spreads to many hospitals and clinics, where we seek to replace antibiotics with aromahoneys, particularly in the field of digestive and respiratory infections. Two hundred and fifty doctors from all over the country attend our lectures in Havana. In the year 2000, one hundred and ninety of them will obtain the first diploma in apitherapy. Without any prompting, the deans from several medicine faculties ask us to go and teach at their universities.

*

Las Terrazzas, a small village some sixty kilometres west of Havana, has been selected to take part in the research. This magnificent site is nestled at the heart of a biosphere nature reserve in which a river with sulphuric water, which is very therapeutic, cascades into emerald-green pools.

The one thousand or so people who live in this privileged environment represent an ideal sample of the Cuban population, and they have always benefited from excellent medical provision. Thanks to the reliable and precise statistics that have been kept, this specific community is going to enable us to set up the first scientific implementation outside of a hospital context. These people are very sensitive to matters of ecology, and many volunteer to replace their usual medical care with aromahoneys, for a period of one year, under the supervision of those doctors we are charged with training. They all get involved in this venture with immense generosity and the feeling that they are taking part in a true march towards progress.

However, the first inhabitant of Las Terrazzas to demonstrate the efficacy of aromahoneys does so by accident. Before the project has even got off the ground, he has been in a hospital in Havana where he has undergone a foot amputation following gangrene. Unfortunately, due to a strain of antibiotic-resistant bacteria, the disease has continued its progress, forcing a second amputation, just below the knee. The poor man is now facing the prospect of a third operation to try and save his life, in the form of an amputation just below the pelvis; this would preclude any possibility of his ever receiving a prosthetic limb at a future date, supposing he is lucky enough to survive.

Prior to operating on him, the surgeon, who is probably convinced that the man is doomed, lets him go home for the weekend. In Las Terrazzas, he bumps into the village doctor, who, seeing the seriousness of his condition, decides to attempt to go for broke, and for two days he applies pure aromahoney dressings straight onto the stump. When the patient gets back to hospital on the Monday morning, the surgeon is astounded. The wound is healing. There is no longer any need to amputate! The story spreads through the village like greased

7. THE HUMANITARIAN SOLUTION

lightning, and it strengthens the inhabitants' confidence in the validity of this medicine. After only a few months, we already know that the first observations are extremely positive.

*

To achieve such good results in such a brief period of time brings immense satisfaction since this type of project, when it passes through international governing bodies, takes an average of seven years to get started, more often than not after the initial enthusiasm has been lost and millions of dollars swallowed up. In order to avoid these pitfalls, we have learnt to rely only on ourselves. Private donors have covered most of the financial side. Some people have without hesitation given their time and called upon their circles of acquaintances in order to ensure the project is developed. Théodore Cherbuliez's personal contribution has been crucial, even if saying so means his modesty has to suffer.

*

We have needed audacity, and also some of the luck that you can trigger if you give it a chance.

This is the case the first time we take sixteen drums of essential oils to Cuba, without any authorisation. My friend Luc, whom I have trained for this new venture, is travelling with me. On the day, at Orly airport we negotiate at the Cubana departures desk in order to obtain free passage for the one hundred and twenty kilos excess baggage. This is granted without too much difficulty by people who prove to be particularly pleasant and understanding.

But the biggest surprise is awaiting us in Havana. Despite our going through customs telling the officials not once but twice that we have goods to declare, they wave us through with a casual wave and without paying any attention to the enormous cartons which have pride of place on our trolleys. Once we are out of the terminal, we laugh as we load our drums onto Adolfo's "company car", a wreck of a Lada which is eighteen years old and has got nearly six hundred thousand kilometres on the clock. Noticing our surprise about the customs, the only explanation he can offer is that of someone who has become blasé and has given up trying to understand the rules of the game, particularly when the coin falls on the right side:- "That's the way it is in Cuba!".

The funniest of all is that Théodore Cherbuliez, who arrives the next day without carrying any goods, is submitted to a thorough search and keeps us waiting over an hour!

Those one hundred litres of organic essential oils, from chemically-assured floral origins, are of pharmaceutical grade. They will enable us to manufacture four thousand doses of antibacterial aromahoneys of perfect quality, which is a must if we are to implement the process on a large scale. Of course, before choosing the essential oils, we have carefully studied the flora on the island, accompanied by forest rangers. We had to be sure that we would at a future date be able to source plants either identical or equivalent to those we use in France, so as to avoid creating a dependency on imported goods.

We are soon reassured on this aspect of the programme. You have to bear in mind that, prior to it being discovered by Christopher Columbus five centuries ago, the island had been covered in a dense tropical forest. In spite of the inevitable deforestation, the vegetation on Cuba is still immensely rich, and those plants which are not available or grow erratically will be cultivated in a rational manner, in close cooperation with rangers and farmers. As a rule we can obtain everything we need simply by asking.

I often give eucalyptus as an example; they are planted in large numbers as they grow very rapidly and their perfectly straight stems are ideal for drying the millions of tobacco leaves that forms the island's prime resource.

It so happens that eucalyptus leaves, which are normally left to rot on the ground once the stems have been stripped, represent a superb raw material for the extraction of an essential oil whose efficacy in the treatment of chest and lung infections is unrivalled.

Forestry and agriculture have therefore become apiculture's indispensable allies, and find a natural place in the therapeutic chain, at the same time regaining a frontline ecological role. The extraction of essential oils allows for the extended use of vegetal material since they can be obtained from plants, leaves, needles or bark. What is less well known is that the by-product of distillation can be used in the preparation of animal feed supplements for cattle.

7. THE HUMANITARIAN SOLUTION

*

Besides its undeniable therapeutic action, green medicine is tri-fold: it is healthy for humans who use it, it is respectful of nature and it is useful for animals.

This is a gentle approach which leaves us to ponder the enormous potential that we, in the west, have squandered. It is true to say that products from the hive and their derivatives can be used for the prevention and treatment of those diseases that threaten our cattle breeding, pig rearing and poultry farming industries. Even if, compared to the cost of lab-produced cures, the cost of 'green' veterinary prophylaxis is higher, this has to be set against the consequences of chemical onslaught, which are unfathomable.

Wouldn't it make sense to devote a little bit more time, and money, to the feeding and care of those creatures we are going to eat, rather than cramming them full with antibiotics, growth hormones and feed manufactured from animal carcasses and dung? Because of our greed, we have transformed animals into terrifying time bombs to which we are exposing our bodies with the tragic prospects both in the short term and the long term that this senseless approach implies. We can observe on a day-to-day basis the helplessness of a Western world that does not know how to repair the damage done to its environment as a result of a mad race that nothing and nobody seem to be able to stop, one that is also making the honeybee one of its victims.

Cultivated areas are sprayed with toxic substances which obviously cannot differentiate between pests and other insects, whatever the manufacturers claim. Honeybees bring back to the hive micro-capsules of insecticides that they have not been able to distinguish from pollen grains, and which constitute mortal poison for their larvae. We use genetic manipulations in an attempt to give plants an artificial 'immune system' – so many dramatic inventions from the sorcerers' apprentices who have, in the name of "progress", caused the loss of half of the honey production in France in 1999.

*

In November 2000, as I arrive in Cuba with Théodore Cherbuliez, Adolfo is waiting for us as usual with his undying smile and his faithful Lada. Everything seems immutable, yet things are changing little by little. In 1998, Canada has gifted the country with a brand new airport and Havana's historic centre, which has recently been listed by Unesco as a world heritage centre, is beginning to be reborn from its own ruins. This week sees the staging in Cuba of the International Green Medicine Congress, and the lobby at our usual hotel, which is usually quiet, is swarming with people.

Adolfo introduces us to a group of young beekeepers from Panama, with whom we soon get into a lively discussion during which I forget my travel weariness. Listening to them, I feel as though I am plunged back into the past. This is because their main concern relates to the sustained aggressiveness amongst their bees, which makes their work hard and very tiresome. Asked whether the bees originate from Africa and whether they are using the famous Langstroth hives, they reply yes on both counts. I am then absolutely delighted to be in a position to explain why, because of their small size, Africanized bees placed in this type of hive are unbearably stressed, hence their aggressive response.

Until they are able to build hives which will be more adapted for these bees' smaller size and different lifestyle, smaller hives both in width and in length, a reduced entrance hole and smaller spaces between the frames, I suggest these passionate beekeepers could add an eleventh frame to the Langstroth hive, which will result in a reduction in the hive volume available and enable the bees to regain some serenity.

*

This is the second time this year that I have been approached about this problem. The previous discussion has taken place in South Africa, where I was in September to prepare for Apimondia 2001.

In the course of my discussions with beekeepers and researchers at the highest level in that country, I have realised that nobody was taking into account the difference in size between European bees and African bees. What had taken me several weeks to discover in the Rwandan forest twenty years earlier has been of no use whatsoever, and the measurements that I had supplied at the time have remained hidden in a drawer somewhere. As suggested by the new Apimondia president, Asger Jorgensen, I am going to have to write up a scientific

7. THE HUMANITARIAN SOLUTION

paper in order to be able to assist the many beekeepers who are battling the same problem in many parts of the world.

The point is, the Africanized honeybee has invaded the whole of the American continent. Not that it set out to do so, but in the same way as slaves many moons ago, it has been imported by men who were seeking profits, and who could only think that by cross-breeding it with local strains they would increase productivity. However, such artificial cross-breeding goes against nature and I am tempted to say constitutes a crime against nature – and nature when deprived of one of its prerogatives always ends up taking revenge.

Moreover, the initial benefits gained by cross-breeding are not passed on to following generations, and man has to carry out more and more complex manipulations in order to retain the advantages thus obtained. This escalation has almost led to serious accidents in the United States, where swarms have been observed attacking cattle or horses and even humans in extreme cases. This behaviour is unthinkable in "natural" bees. But man is capable of sacrificing anything on the altar of profit.

The ultimate stage of this rapacity has been reached in Canada, where beekeepers had got into the habit of culling their bees at the end of the summer season for economic reasons. It was more worthwhile for them to buy cheap colonies from the US every year and to start over from scratch rather than suffer the high level of honey consumption required by bees over the winter, and the usual spring losses.

Then a few years ago they started overwintering bees in temperature-controlled sheds at between minus five and plus five degrees, the optimal temperature for a reasonable honey consumption and an easy spring kick-start. Was this change of method due to a sudden realisation about their scornful behaviour towards such a generous animal? Only partly. The threat of varroa, introduced to the neighbouring United States, has forced them to close their borders to the importation of bee colonies, thereby encouraging a return to a respectful attitude towards nature.

*

Varroa is a dreaded mite, which resides with some bees in China and India that have learnt to adapt to it and to live with it. Within a few years, due to some of the cross-breeding programmes that are very fashionable in "modern" beekeeping, the mite has spread all over the world at an alarming rate and it has decimated more than half of the domestic and wild honeybees which haven't had time to adapt or develop an efficient defence mechanism against the onslaught of this alien species.

*

I remember a beekeeper in Serres, in the High Alps district in France. During the course of my studies he had come to talk to us about his work and his ideas, which were going against the current thinking and had really impressed me.

He was battling against the concept of industrial beekeeping and the notion of profitability at any cost: he was refusing to use antibiotics in his hives and was warning, ten years before the appearance of varroa, against the madness of cross-breeding supposed to increase productivity. He, on the other hand, was advocating breed specificity, explaining how one strain is perfectly adapted to its environment and able to resist its predators. He said we could just about give natural selection a helping hand in order to improve upon the qualities of a local strain; but it had to be first and foremost for its own benefit, and not to serve man's interests, man being the worst of predators with his unbridled appetite.

At a time when we were not allowed to mention "organic" farming within the college, this man had struck me as a visionary and a humanitarian: a real "bee shepherd".

History has proved me right, but the lesson has not been understood. We are still trying to eradicate varroa mites by using chemicals which have been developed by the same labs that produce millions of pills for human use, whereas all you would need to do is go into forests and study wild colonies which have become varroa-resistant. Let's be humble. Let's observe how nature is capable of evolving resistant strains and to solve the problem without man's "help" since nature could very well do without man, whereas the reverse is not true.

Nature alone can grasp the notion of timelessness and impermanence, can differentiate between what is essential and what is mere unimportant detail. Notions of time and space are not the same. Nature respects the rhythm of both. Its transformations occur on a scale that

7. THE HUMANITARIAN SOLUTION

we find hard to accept and that frighten us, because it reminds us of how ephemeral we are. We also have suicidal tendencies, because each and every act of aggression against nature gets turned back against us day after day. We have forgotten the laws of harmony which should dictate our conduct, and we have lost our knowledge of what is universal – to which honeybees always bring us back.

*

I am once again reminded of all that this week, as I go back to see an apiary of Apis Mellipona, the sacred bee of the Mayas, which is only found in Central America and which I have discovered during my second trip to Cuba.

Since it does not possess a system capable of regulating the temperature within the hive, this bee requires constant temperatures and a climate that remains the same all year round. It uses a mixture of wax and mud to fashion little pyramid-shaped pots which it piles on top of one another, storing the honey horizontally in a departure from what other bees do. This bee is wonderfully docile, and the only one of the species that never stings... because it doesn't have a stinger. It is also the only bee with blue eyes. And as luck would have it, it produces tiny quantities of a honey which nevertheless has specific therapeutic properties that enable us to prepare excellent eye drops.

Once again I feel a strong emotion at the sight of this unique bee species and at the immense kindness of the beekeeper, a farmer who, strangely, also has blue eyes and who has invited us to come back one day and accompany him on a trip to observe forest mellipona. Before we leave he even checks with Adolfo whether I would accept his present of a bottle of this very rare honey. He says it as if it was him who would be honoured! I accept, on condition that he allows me to buy some pollen from him. That way the exchange is a fair one.

*

At our first works meeting in Havana I am awaiting the results from the clinical tests with barely concealed anticipation. For six months, the team at the Finlay Institute, under Doctor Guillermo Prodo, has been treating cases of general infection (septicaemia) and of chest and lung infections (pneumonia, bronchopneumonia, bronchial asthma) with my aroma-honeys.

The official figures that Guillermo announces, smiling widely, are astonishing. Out of more than a thousand cases, the success rate is one hundred per cent! Théo and I look at each other, we are delirious with joy... and immediately worried. We can already foresee how the international scientific community's eyebrows are going to be raised in the face of a success that some will find too good to be true. Yet...

We play devil's advocate, we ply Guillermo with trick questions and we ask him to give a precise account of his working methods. He responds with serenity. Everything is strictly in accordance with the protocols. The graphs showing the disappearance of various symptoms (coughs, fever, expectorations) over ten days are beyond any doubt. The trials confirm categorically the powers of this new "medicine" compared to antibiotics, be it as far as duration of the infection is concerned, or stem resistance, or chronicity, or recrudescence.

The first trials on wound-healing propo-honey, which have been started at a later date, and cannot therefore be included in the statistics, also already show a level of efficacy markedly superior to that of chemical products. The study is now going to be extended to include conditions affecting the digestive system. After what we have just heard, I am entirely confident.

What we already knew from our own experience, and which has now been confirmed scientifically, is that patients respond perfectly to the treatment and that there are no negative side effects whatsoever. What we also know, but will be harder to prove, is that there are some side effects, but that they are positive side effects and that they contribute greatly to the patient's rapid recovery. I stand up and I clasp Guillermo in a bear-hug. This is one of the most beautiful days of my life.

On the following Thursday, in the course of the Green Medicine Congress, we present our results to a crowded room. This is a very moving moment. For the first time I see the young doctors, whom we have been training for two years, wearing suits and ties, and laying out their arguments with self-assurance despite their stage fright. Amongst the public, interest is growing by the minute. Each participant is aware that he or she is witnessing the birth of a "discovery" – and I choose my words carefully – which is comparable to that of antibiotics. The

7. THE HUMANITARIAN SOLUTION

audience's deep silence is impressive.

Having dealt with the numbers in their implacable rigour, the graphs, the statistics and detailed explanations by various members of his team, Guillermo offers to show a video report about two of their patients, Manuel and Sergio, two MS sufferers whom they have been treating for several months with apipuncture. Manuel's smiling account ends with the most beautiful turn of phrase that I have heard so far: "I am now feeling much better thanks to the honeybee's kiss."

Sergio, whom I had met when he first arrived in the department, was practically in a coma. His illness, which had already made an invalid of him, had been seriously worsened by the Interferon B treatment that he had received when the doctors were still regarding it as an efficient weapon in their armoury. Today he still finds it difficult to talk, but he has regained all his faculties. The emotional climax is reached when he stands up from his chair and slowly walks across the room in front of the camera.

The lights come back on. We all have a lump in our throats and we are all misty-eyed. A man stands up and asks Guillermo to pass him the microphone. He is a professor of neurology and at the head of the fight against multiple sclerosis in Cuba, and we know him well from our original confrontation when we introduced our initial work, to which he was fiercely hostile. We await his reaction with some anxiety. Very soon, despite my very basic knowledge of Spanish, I realise that he has changed his mind radically, and that he has become a strong defender of our cause. He congratulates us on the progress we have achieved, he acknowledges the limitations of standard medicine, although he sponsors it himself in the treatment of some conditions, and he encourages his colleagues to open their minds to these methods which, he thinks, carry great hope. He has gone to the trouble of studying the way bee venom operates, and he has understood the advantages that could be derived for patients, whose interests are paramount.

I can't believe my ears. When he has finished speaking and has been rewarded with a burst of applause, I go and thank him heartily.

We leave the conference hall with our heads in the clouds. My only regret is that members of the apitherapy commission, who have got involved body and soul in the project from the very beginning, are not here to share this extraordinary moment. After so many battles, this recognition is a veritable consecration, even though we have to bear in mind that it is not the crowning glory of our endeavour but rather the promise of a grand departure.

*

Good news can hide bad news. In the evening we get together at Guillermo's dispensary, where, despite their meagre means, they have organised a little party for my birthday. This kind gesture is very touching and goes straight to my heart. Doctor Jorge Menendez Hernandez, who is Conchita's right arm, gives me the best present by announcing that the Finlay Institute will from now on employ five full timers to oversee the development of clinical trials: a biologist, an immunologist, a pharmacist, an epidemiologist and a statistician. And that is not all. Jorge also explains that the first trials on the antiviral remedies that I have been working on, still based on products from the hive, are going to commence thanks to the arrival of this new team.

After the official announcement by the Ministries for Health and Agriculture, at the beginning of the year, that apitherapy has been declared of national interest and that a three-year plan had been established to develop it, we have passed another crucial milestone. This is evidence that the government is pulling out all the stops to assist the project. It has to be said that we are in the process of revolutionising medical care from a therapeutic point of view since we are about to replace up to seventy per cent of chemical medicines with green pharmacopeia. Furthermore, our method also blows economic rules to smithereens. Who in the West could conceive of a full two-week treatment to defeat once and for all a case of pneumonia with secondary infection with an overall cost of ... ONE dollar?

The next evening, on the planc home, sleep eludes me, due to a happiness overdose. After years of efforts and of renewed efforts, I feel that the fruit of our endeavours is coming to maturity and that the future is at last beginning to take shape. I look back to those long hours spent waiting around in offices, trying to defeat the inherent inertia of all those administrations whose bureaucracy seems to have only one aim, that of self-preservation. "I exist, therefore I am", and vice-versa.

I can still hear those endless discussions about minute details during

7. THE HUMANITARIAN SOLUTION

which we would lose sight of the essential. I recall the wave of anger which assailed me on two occasions, when I thought nothing was progressing and I threatened never to come back, although deep down I knew full well that I wouldn't carry it through. So many people and so many events mean that I have become attached to this country in the course of a few years.

I can still see, at the end of a Sunday dinner with some officials whose opinion was vital for the future of our project, Théodore Cherbuliez standing up and pronouncing with great audacity the few premonitory words which I am convinced weighed heavily in the final decision: "What we are proposing is the setting up of tomorrow's medicine , which will preserve nature as well as present and future generations. The name for this change of direction in medicine is a word which is close to every Cuban's heart: revolution."

8. Soldiering On...

The Cuban adventure will last for some ten years, punctuated by peaks of immense satisfaction and undeniable signs of progress, which unfortunately get slowed down by the clumsiness inherent in a system that will end up eroding our initial enthusiasm.

Between October 2001 and October 2002, we return to Las Terrazzas to carry out an in-depth study on the therapeutic benefits in primary care of using two aroma-honey formulations with anti-microbial properties and one propo-honey formulation with antiseptic and wound-healing properties. The team comprises eight doctors, of whom three are from the Finlay Institute and the other five are practitioners from the village clinic.

As early as May 2001 our encounters with the village inhabitants bear fruit. The vast majority of the residents are in favour of supporting a project such as ours. They are aware of what is at stake and of the possible fallout that such a program can trigger for other humanitarian projects not only in Cuba but also in the rest of the world. The project aims to corroborate the studies and results previously obtained within hospitals. The group, which consists of more than 1,000 villagers living in this biosphere natural park, will be all the more representative in that from a health point of view they have been followed for many years, and there exist solid statistical sets of data.

*

The first stage consists in training the medical team in all the apitherapy techniques which are used, mostly in clinical applications where there is a particular requirement for wound healing. We also teach them the protocols for treating broncho-pulmonary infections, and other infections, using aroma-honeys. We are careful not to use any essential oils with unwanted side-effects, apart from the essential oil from Thymus vulgaris whose thymol has a toxic effect on the liver. Although the dosage at which we operate is well below the toxicity level, it is recommended that particular care should be taken with patients suffering from chronic or acute liver conditions, even if the treatment's dosage level is between forty and sixty times lower than that of the toxic dosage.

The addition of propolis and Basilicum essential oil, which are both liver protectors, reduces the level of toxicity and thus increases the safety margin. Moreover, tests carried out on mice have shown that in order to show significant toxicity it would take a level 400 times greater than the therapeutic dosage we prescribe.

The all-purpose aroma-honey is used as a broad spectrum antibiotic against all stomach complaints, gingivitis, vaginal infections, chronic vaginal infections, urinary infections, bacterial conjunctivitis, pyoderma gangrenosum and lymphangititis cases.

The broncho-pulmonary aroma-honey is used against rhinitis, pharyngitis, rhino-pharyngitis, the common cold and more complex colds with associated bacterial infections, acute bronchitis, acute chronic bronchitis, sinusitis, ear infections and bronchial asthma attacks.

The dosage is three times a day for the first week, ie 15g a day for patients weighing less than forty kilos, 30g a day for those between forty and a hundred kilos, and 45g a day for those weighing more than a hundred kilos. The dosage is reduced by half for the second week.

Propo-honey, with its antiseptic and wound-healing properties, is used for the treatment of infections due to injuries or burns. The product is applied every day and covered with sterile gauze for the first two weeks, then every other day until complete cicatrisation.

The results are perfectly in accordance with our most optimistic predictions.

For the first two weeks of treatment, the group treated with the all-purpose aroma-honey achieves a rate of 82% complete cure. Only one patient, with a urinary infection, fails to get better during the two-week period. Another two, suffering from gingivitis and periodontal diseases, show an improvement in their symptoms but not a complete healing before the end of the trial period.

The efficacy of the all-purpose aroma-honey manifests itself

8. SOLDIERING ON

between the 7th and 21st days of treatment, depending on the pathology and on the patient's response to the product. Side effects vary. They range from simple nausea to gastro-intestinal problems, with sometimes a general feeling of not being well, but these symptoms usually disappear between the third and sixth day of treatment and they do not return.

Amongst the group treated with the broncho-pulmonary aroma-honey, we obtain a rate of 88% cure during the first two weeks' treatment, whatever the pathology had been.

As far as the group treated with the propo-honey is concerned, we reach an efficacy rate of 95% with a total absence of side effects apart from one case of itching or skin irritation at the time of the product being applied. This only goes to confirm to us that the blood flow is activated and that cellular division is taking place within the damaged tissue when placed in contact with the propo-honey, which acts as a growth agent for the granulating tissue as soon as it comes into contact with the epithelial cells. This confirms the results obtained by our friend Bernard Descottes in Limoges.

Moreover, a case of ulcer with staphylococcal bacterial complications and a case of infected wound are treated with a combination of propo-honey and all-purpose honey, which achieves healing within less than two weeks.

*

On the whole, we can therefore claim that the treatments we have used have been efficient, well received by the patients, and most importantly there have not been any incidences of toxicity.

It is also important to note that diagnosis has been achieved without the help of any X-rays or invasive techniques such as would be required for sampling tests.

The villagers are unanimous when it comes to the improvement brought to their quality of life, and they come to us completely aware of the hope that their experiences will engender.

*

On the strength of the extremely positive conclusions from the experiments at Las Terrazzas, we offer to take on cases of extreme antibiotic-resistant infections. Despite the scale of the problem, it will take us several months of administrative procedures to win the day. Numerous presentations and scientific presentations are required in order to convince the other departments, in particular the medical ethics committee, to accept this project. Indeed, even in extreme cases, using the population as guinea pigs was out of the question. Eventually, through perseverance and against the opinion of some heads of clinics fiercely hostile to our integration, we join the Frank Pais hospital in Havana, from which foreigners are in theory totally banned.

We are entrusted with a department which has been created to gather together all the antibiotic-resistant orthopaedic cases deemed incurable by all the other hospitals in the country, who see amputation as the only ultimate solution for such extreme cases.

*

For a period of four years, we are going to be leading a study on the antibiotic and healing properties of the combination of what we call proparomiel (propolis, essential oils and honey). During the course of this study we will have to battle against administrative red tape and the deep-rooted habits amongst nurses, which we will "challenge" a little, in particular in order to impose a twice-daily change of dressings for some patients.

During this time, thanks to the remarkable initial results, and to the speed achieved in healing, all of Cuba's hopeless cases end up in our department, since the medical authorities consider that we can't do these patients any harm seeing that they are doomed.

Isassi's wonderful experience, among other successes, was one we shared. He is a man in his sixties who has been suffering with a crippling infection in his femur for over five years, and who will only regain full use of his leg after more than a year under our treatment.

Following three months of pre-op treatment, when he is given a daily dose of nine capsules, as well as a deep cleansing of the infected area in order to sanitize the surrounding soft tissue, Doctor Franco Feraboli, who is a member of the Apitherapy Commission, comes over to carry out the operation and to teach his fellow surgeons how to use apitherapy within the operating block.

Thus they discover how to clean a wound using honey vinegar and

8. SOLDIERING ON

then, after the affected bone has been cleansed, how to use raw honey as a detergent, and finally they learn about injecting proparomiel straight into the bone in order to eradicate the infection.

*

In total our study extends to 150 patients presenting with various chronic multi-resistant bone tissue and soft tissue infections, which are more often than not hospital-acquired conditions.

Chronic musculoskeletal, cardiovascular and neurological infections are quite common in orthopaedic surgery, and they are the most difficult to treat among septic incidences. Surgery does not always allow for the total eradication of infection, in particular for patients equipped with artificial limbs.

Hospital-acquired infections are particularly persistent in that they are both frequent and resistant to treatment. In France, where they affect around 800,000 people, they cause some five thousand deaths each year and they lead to large numbers of amputations. The lengthy periods of incapacity that they trigger, as well as their after effects, have a serious impact on the patients' quality of life and on the whole of society. Moreover, they engender suspicion towards hospitals and the quality of treatment offered, thus acting against medicine as a whole.

In the United States, septicaemia and pneumonia, the two most common hospital-acquired infections, kill nearly 50,000 people each year and their treatment has cost eight billion dollars in 2006!

What are the causes of this disaster? Carelessness within the cleaning and disinfection processes in hospital buildings, defective sterilisation of instruments, and even, as incredible as it may seem in our day and age, simple bad hand-hygiene amongst medical staff.

Lastly and foremost, we have seen an increased level of resistance within bacterial strains to those precious antibiotics which, if one were to believe the medicine of the nineteen fifties, were going to rid us forever of the scourge that are infections. Unfortunately, whereas in 1942, 10,000 units of penicillin a day for four days were sufficient to cure a case of Type A streptococcal pneumonia, the same infection is, fifty years later, capable of resisting a course of 25million units per day for eight days! Yet, it is estimated that better prevention could reduce such infections by 20% to 30%!

The most common strain to be found in these infections is, in more than 60% of cases, Staphylococcus aureus. It is often found associated with negative Gram bacillus, the latter being involved in more than 30% of the cases that are reported in scientific publications.

The use of antibiotics for lengthy periods is responsible for allergic reactions, for the increase of bacterial resistance, and for the lowering of immunity and medicine-induced gastro-enteritis. Furthermore, microbial capacity for implantation in bone tissue has also been modified.

The above factors can explain the failure of treatments in the short and medium term. In the United States, there are more than one million cases every year of infections due to hospital germs. Despite the large variety of forms of resistance and the increasing number of their harmful effects, antibiotic consumption is constantly on the increase.

*

"Once you've got a bone infection, you've got it for good." This old saying which is still current within orthopaedic departments goes a long way to show how bone infections are still very difficult to put right.

It is with a view to bringing a solution to this problem that Professor Cherbuliez and I have developed proparomiel, which is composed of standardized natural products such as honey, propolis extracts and essential oils obtained by distillation in water vapour of known medicinal plants. Each of these components contains natural antimicrobial properties. Their therapeutic performance is supported by a large body of published university work.

Based on positive results observed during a previous study, we had suggested we could, for the first time in Cuba, apply this product to hospital-acquired infections.

The results from studies on antibacterial activity in vitro and toxicity in vivo, which have been carried out at the Finlay Institute in Havana as well as by a Belgian laboratory in collaboration with a Walloon university, have demonstrated the absence of toxicity for the dosage used, as well as the efficacy of propo-aroma-honey as a broad-spectrum natural antibacterial substance. Moreover, the use of proparomiel in association with antibiotics is efficient against a large number of multi-resistant bacteria.

Two groups have been set up.

The 120 patients in group A have been treated with a proparomiel alongside a chemical antibiotic treatment administered orally, intramuscularly and intravenously.

The 30 patients in group B, who are allergic to antibiotics, have been treated with the proparomiel only.

The results which had been obtained on these 150 patients during the twelve months prior to the study will act as a control and point of comparison. They have all received intermittent antibiotic treatments ranging in duration from one to forty years, with recurring infections that have become more and more difficult to treat.

The antibiotics for group A have been prescribed by the orthopaedic surgeon and the department doctor, after they have had the results of the lab tests confirmed. The latter have been carried out in the microbiology lab at the teaching hospital. Samples have been taken from patients every 15 days at the start of the study and subsequently.

On surface wounds the proparomiel salve has been used at a 3.3% concentration in local treatment: daily topical application on ulcers and surface lesions, which have been cleaned up with a saline solution before the wounds are dressed with sterile gauze.

A 1.1% proparomiel preparation is injected once a day straight into deep wounds and fistulas, again after saline cleansing. The area around the wound or fistula is massaged lightly before and during instillation so as to stimulate blood flow and ensure a homogenous delivery and good absorption of the product.

In some cases, two external applications have been applied to patients suffering from significant purulent secretions.

Additionally, all patients have taken orally twice daily a teaspoon of 2% proparomiel in the form of a syrup.

*

90 patients were suffering from osteomyelitis bone infection. This chronic infection can, if left untreated, persist intermittently for years. 72 of these cases were due to Staphylococcus aureus and 48 were methycilline resistant. The other cases comprised 24 chronic infected ulcers with various etiologies, 21 infected surgical open wounds, 9 ulcers

due to malum perforans pedis, and 6 cases of infected pressure ulcers.

Biopsies have shown the predominance of Staphylococcus aureus in chronic infections in 96 of the patients. Other resistant germs have also been isolated and identified, but they are present in lower percentages: Pseudomona aeruginosa in 19 cases, Enterobacter aglomerans in 8 cases, Proteus mirabilis in 3 cases. And, for the 24 remaining cases, we have found a combination of Staphylococcus aureus with other germs such as Escherichia coli (8), Serratia sp (10) and Pseudomona aeruginosa (6).

These results agree with those reported in various scientific publications, which indicate that more than 60% of the germs found in infections are due to the presence of Staphylococcus aureus and that they can be associated with negative Gram bacilli, such as Pseudomonas aeruginosa and Escherichia coli among others.

Group B has shown that the treatment had an antibacterial, anti-inflammatory and reparative action on damaged tissue similar to that in group A, but with a faster response to treatment, emphasized by a more rapid disappearance of the signs of infection.

Within group B, at day fifteen of the treatment, only 15% of patients were still in need of fresh dressings three times a day, whereas the figure was 45% in group A.

Similar results have been obtained for other clinical criteria: inflammation, pain, redness and raised temperature around the wound, with group B showing a quicker response than group A.

These results can be explained by invoking a diminished response from an immune system that has been submitted to antibiotic treatments, but also by an increase in resistance to bacterial strains from patients who are regularly treated with antibiotics.

As far as body temperature is concerned, it is important to note that, because of its stimulating effect on immune responses, proparomiel can in some patients bring about an increase in symptomatology, a general feeling of being unwell and a raised temperature between days 3 and 5 of the treatment. These symptoms disappear after the first week of treatment.

Proparomiel has been able to bring about a solution, both at a systemic and local level, from the initial three days of treatment, thus increasing patients' quality of life, patients who had often lost faith in

8. SOLDIERING ON

medical practice and abandoned hope of ever recovering and resuming normal life.

All cases of chronic ulcers, in both groups, have been cured within a time span of between 21 and 90 days' treatment. Ulcers due to malum perforans pedis have required nine months. Those with a diagnosis of bone infection have needed 4 to 24 months. The only recurrence has happened in the case of an infected pressure ulcer, one year after healing. Infected surgical wounds have required around fifteen months to heal.

*

Out of the 90 cases of bone infection, 66 are considered to be healed. The other 24 have shown distinct improvements up to the point of regaining the ability to walk, even though on X-rays they still presented with signs of infection in the bone two years after the start of the treatment. This is hardly surprising if you think that some of these conditions had been present for five years and that the patients in question had completely lost the use of their legs prior to receiving our treatment. Finally, nine amputations which had been deemed inevitable have been avoided.

Two years on from the end of the study, no recurrence has been reported.

*

With a final rate of cure of 88%, it can be said that proparomiel is efficient in the fight against pathologies engendered by multi-resistant bacteria. Moreover, these tests demonstrate that there has been no adverse reaction to the combining of antibiotics with proparomiel, and that it does not act any better than proparomiel on its own.

This is the reason why, two years later, proparomiel is officially registered in Cuba as a licensed medicine. In all, five products will receive this supreme accolade: one antiviral, one all-round antibacterial, one broncho-pulmonary anti-infectious, one ENT (ear nose and throat) anti-infectious and one wound-healing product.

It has taken two whole years spent following never-ending procedures in order to put together the case files, and all that despite using computers that kept breaking down and photocopiers without paper!

At about the same time, Théodore Cherbuliez and I get to meet Professor Juan Ramos, head of the serious burns unit at the Calixto Garcia teaching hospital in Havana. Due to the lack of French-Spanish interpreters, my wife Barbara, who is perfectly bi-lingual, has offered to take charge of translating our conversations.

At the hospital, we are told that the lift is temporarily out of service – which in Cuba means that it hasn't worked since 1960 – and we walk up the six floors to reach the department.

Once there, we discover that Cuban doctors use a technique which is slightly at odds with our own methods. They soak the first dressing in a solution of honey and propolis prior to applying it to the burnt area, and they remove it 24 hours later to apply a fresh dressing which they then leave in situ, whilst re-soaking it with the same mixture every day.

A patient comes towards us. She had been admitted the day before with serious burns from her neck to her navel area. She is invited to sit down on a stainless steel table, and the nurse starts to remove the dressing unceremoniously. She isn't using any saline solution in order to facilitate the process, instead yanking the dressing off as though it was a mere band-aid, making the patient's eyes water, although she remains heroically stoical. My wife, who is not accustomed to witnessing this sort of thing, promptly faints, only to be immediately surrounded by a group of bemused medics who thereby leave the burns patient to her own devices!

The same will happen later on to our Cuban interpreter as we make our way through the waiting room of the children's burns clinic. In order to avoid this type of problem, we eventually recruit a pharmacist who specialises in natural remedies, Doctor Liena Hernandez, to be our interpreter during hospital visits. Thanks to her work, at the Franck Pais hospital among others, she will become a member of the apitherapy commission a few years later.

Doctor Juan Ramos will subsequently publish the results of many studies to attest to the efficiency of the burns treatment and to the undeniable improvement of honey-healed wounds, thereby confirming the accuracy of the work carried out in France by Bernard Descottes, as

8. SOLDIERING ON

well as that undertaken by Peter Mullan in New Zealand and Australia.

*

Between 2002 and 2005 we organize three international congresses at Havana's university teaching hospital, during which Théodore Cherbuliez, all the members of the apitherapy commission and myself give lectures which are each time attended by three hundred and fifty participants from some twenty different nations, mostly from Central and South America but also from Canada, the United States, Russia and Europe. To gather together eleven apitherapy teachers from all over the world is in itself a tour de force, but to get them to teach in a complementary way is like a miracle. Each is intent on speaking about his own research and its results, even when those are off-subject and far removed from the course these experts have been called upon to deliver.

*

In total, we train around five hundred doctors and pharmacists, as well as some thirty biologists and a large number of nurses. More and more hospital departments are using products from the hive and their various combinations as therapeutic solutions.

This body of work will give rise to a number of publications, mostly in Latin America where Cuban medicine enjoys an excellent reputation.

*

As the saying goes, everything seemed to be going for the best in the best of worlds, but two events were to precipitate the end of our beautiful adventure.

First of all we see the departure – or rather the escape – for Mexico, by the doctor in charge of studying the effects of bee venom in the fight against multiple sclerosis. This will signal the death knell of this otherwise promising work, which is automatically struck off Cuban medicine at the same time as the name of its director is removed.

Then, a little while later, a decision made by the Ministry of Finance falls upon us, and it is without appeal. It has been decided that, in order to favour the exportation of Cuban honey, which is an important source of currency, the use of this precious product as either foodstuff or for medical purposes is forbidden on the island from now on.

*

Not only have the state bureaucrats taken no account of the therapeutic and humanitarian benefits, which should have been at the forefront of their thinking, but they have also omitted to remember that apitherapy offered important savings, since it was enabling Cuba to reduce its imports of chemical medicines, which enable the pharmaceutical industry to get rich, a potent symbol of capitalism, against which they fight so hard!

Paradoxically, it is thanks to the work of Cuban doctors who have been sent by their own government to work in various Latin American countries that there is a widespread use of practices which have officially today all but disappeared.

For his part, our friend Adolfo continues to supply hospitals on the sly and, if apitherapy is still alive in Cuba, we have to be grateful for the tenacity and courage of men and women like him, of all the people trained over the years, and for a population that sought to find natural solutions for their health, and in particular from apitherapy products.

The medical teams who have taken part in this adventure, the patients and their families, whom we have followed for all those years, all have brought us moments of such happiness that they are forever engraved on our memory.

But most of all we have the island's bees to thank, those bees sacred to Cubans, and even more so for all those people who have during this time been treated with the fabulous substances which they are relentlessly producing.

er
8. SOLDIERING ON

9. A Pharmacopeia Direct from the Hive

As I showed at the beginning of the book, the hive is a fantastic laboratory within which bees, since time immemorial, have been producing medicines indispensable for man's health.

Honey.

This is the leading product and it has always been used for its nutritious, healing and spiritual properties. It results from the blending together of the animal and the vegetal and is therefore a substance with strong energising powers. The bees forage for flower nectar, which contains sugars, water, vitamins and minerals. Nectar is a concentrated form of processed sap. In order for it to become honey, this nectar is passed around by the bees from tongue to tongue until a water concentration of around 50% is reached; it is then stored within the hive and matures through evaporation until its water content drops to approximately 18%.

The many types of honey available all contain roughly the same percentages of sugars. What differentiates them in respect of scent, taste, appearance and therapeutic properties is the various contents of vitamins, minerals, organic acids, enzymes and essential oils.

Honey contains 75% to 80% carbohydrates as follows:-

Fructose +/- 35%
Glucose +/- 32%
Maltose +/- 4%
Sucrose +/- 2%

Fructose and glucose are readily digestible, whereas industrially-produced sucrose has to be transformed. Honey can be said to be pre-digested as bees have, with their saliva and the help of an enzyme called invertase, transformed sucrose into so-called 'inverted' sugar. This enzyme is very sensitive to heat and is destroyed at temperatures above 45°. Honey should therefore never be heated up.

Whereas glucose provides a source of instantly available energy, fructose is stored in the liver as starch, and makes up our energy stocks, which will enable us, amongst other things, to respond to stress.

Moreover, honey prevents hypoglycaemia which can be occasioned by the consumption of industrial sugar, and it is singularly compatible with some forms of diabetes.

With the exception of vitamin A, honey contains almost all known vitamins, some of them at trace levels. 1.5% to 2% of its contents is made up of trace elements and minerals whose effects combine with those of vitamins: calcium, magnesium, phosphorus, potassium, copper, iron, chlorine, silica, sulphur, manganese and sodium, among others.

It is interesting to note that a study carried out by Germans in the Ruhr Valley, one of the country's most polluted areas, has shown that bees were carefully selecting those components that contained the least amounts of toxic heavy metals, and that the honeys harvested there had a very low poison content. By preserving their own health, the bees manufacture the purest of products, even given the worst circumstances, thereby protecting us too.

*

Honey contains organic acids such as gluconic acid, citric acid, acetic acid and phosphoric acid which give it a pH between 3.5 and 5.5. It also contains numerous enzymes, the main ones being alpha amylase and beta amylase, glucose invertase and glucose oxidase.

Some pollen is present, albeit at a very low percentage, and this characteristic enables the floral origin of honey to be ascertained.

Honey also contains essential oils, in quantities and concentrations that vary according to the floral origin. These are of primordial importance both from a gustative and from a therapeutic point of view.

*

Water represents between 17% and 20% of honey's total weight. It is

9. A PHARMACOPEIA DIRECT FROM THE HIVE

known that water originating from sap is ionised and that it is easily absorbed and circulated throughout the body (birch sap for instance).

Depending on their floral origin, different honeys will have various therapeutic effects on all of the human body: growth, immune system, respiratory system, digestive system. They also act as healing agents on skin for normal wounds, infected wounds and burns.

Pollen.

Pollen is a flower's "sperm". It is composed of microscopic grains which the honeybee gathers by rolling and rubbing in the flowers. The grains cling to her hairs, in particular to those on her abdomen.

Thanks to the brushes and combs that equip her hind legs, the bee is able to gather these grains together and, using a mixture of saliva and nectar, she fashions little pollen balls that she will then carry in her purpose-built pollen baskets, also situated on her hind legs. Back at the hive, the pollen loads are stored for a few days. Due to fermentation, they transform into what is known as bee-bread, which will be used to feed larvae and young bees.

During their constant quest for pollen, insects carry it from flower to flower, thereby fertilizing the plants they visit. This is called pollinisation.

*

Pollen is extremely rich in amino acids. 100 grams of this vegetable "steak" is equivalent to the protein content of 7 eggs or 500 grams of beef meat.

It comprises:-

Water: between 11% and 18% in the case of fresh pollen, and between 4% and 5% for dry pollen.

Amino-acids: our bodies contain between 20 and 22 of these, and in pollen we find the 8 essential amino-acids: cysteine, isoleucine, leucine, glycine, methionine, phenylalanine, tryptophan and tyrosine.

Other nitrogenous products such as peptones, globulins, DNA and RNA.

Hydrocarbons: glucose, fructose, sucrose, pentosan, dextrose, starch, cellulose, pollenine.

Lipids: fatty acids, mostly unsaturated, lecithin, good cholesterol, pre-prostaglandins

Enzymes: phosphatise, catalase, cozymase, amylase, invertase, persine, trypsine, lipase. Enzymes act as catalysts. They are essential for a large number of metabolic processes.

Minerals and trace elements; it is one of nature's richest source of these elements. Pollen's numerous constituents, as well as their levels, mean that it has a therapeutic action that goes well beyond that of a simple foodstuff.

Vitamins: Provitamin A, vitamins from the B group as well as Vitamins C, D and E. Pollen contains twenty times more carotene than carrots do.

Growth hormones.

Natural ferments which encourage probiotic activity and replenish intestinal flora.

Antibacterial substances which are particularly efficient in the treatment of gastro-intestinal complaints and colibacillocis.

Many pigments.

*

The therapeutic action of pollen can be applied to any part of the body, but it is particularly suitable for conditions affecting the digestive system and urinary tract, as well as for the prevention of cardio-vascular diseases. Paradoxically, pollen is also recommended in the treatment of allergies that are generally imputed to it.

Allergies and natural desensitization.

Are allergies this century's new disease? Despite the expression being somewhat debased, it is true that this type of disorder sits on the "hit parade" alongside back-pain and stress, other pathologies which are typical of the modern world.

In this type of disorder, heredity and biology play an appreciable role, but it is now known that behaviour and environment, in the widest sense of the term, also have an important impact on the phenomenon. We increasingly question the obsession with hygiene within our society, which leads us to want to keep newborn babies in quasi-sterile surroundings, or later on, to stop children rolling around in the sand

9. A PHARMACOPEIA DIRECT FROM THE HIVE

pit. Deprived of bacteria and other micro-organisms against which it would be fighting, the immune system "invents" enemies in order to preserve its defence mechanisms. Thereby cat or rabbit or hamster fur, dust, strawberries, kiwi fruit, eggs or peanuts defy all logic to become enemies for thousands of children, for whom life will become strewn with death traps. If we include the adverse effects of chemical pollution, both external and internal, which disrupt our hormonal system, we can soon understand why allergies have become one of the worst scourges of modern times.

According to scientific definition, type I allergy is a quasi-immediate exaggerated immunological response linked to an abnormal production of immunoglobulin E (IgE). Type II hyper-sensibility is also known as cytotoxicity. It starts 4 to 6 hours after contact with the allergen. It can be observed when an antibody (immunoglobulin G) reacts with an antigen that has been absorbed through a cellular membrane, or with one of its natural constituents. Atopic syndrome is the name given to the genetic pre-disposition to develop such reactions.

So, an allergy is an excessive reaction by the immune system following exposure to a substance generally foreign to the body.

To put it more simply, it is an individual's abnormal reaction to a substance which is a priori harmless but which is identified by the body as a potential danger against which it deploys a whole panoply of defences.

*

The immune system's role is to defend the body against any foreign aggression. To that effect, it produces antibodies (immunoglobulin) tasked with creating an immune response to intruders. In the case of allergies, this defence mechanism oversteps its role and considers as harmful some substances which are not, or should not be, harmful. Allergic reactions are the result of such derangement, in which histamine plays a crucial role.

Histamine is a chemical mediator which, when released during hypersensitivity episodes, stimulates the secretion of gastric juices and hydrochloric acid, the relaxation of artery walls, contraction of bronchial tubes and intestinal muscles, and an acceleration of the heart's beat. Histamine is responsible for vasodilatation and oedema, for anaphylactic shock, for inflammation and for rashes.

Once the process has been started, it is not always easy to "re-educate" the immune system. Depending on the severity of the reaction, there are different types of treatment available. Antihistamines, steroids, broncho-dilators and adrenalin are the most commonly used protocols. Although these substances are necessary in cases of emergency, they are only a stop-gap solution which, although essential, is not sufficient in the long term. Many an allergy sufferer, having used these chemical compounds, has seen the necessity to increase the dosage year on year, only to "logically" come to resort to taking cortisone, with its attendant negative side effects, without being able to see a possible end to the problem, leading to an infernal downward spiral.

The real treatment, the one that makes for the re-programming of our defences and an exit from the process, is achieved through auto-vaccination, desensitization, a change in feeding habits, even acupuncture and osteopathy.

Products from the hive fit in perfectly with this philosophy of a medicine that respects people and respects life.

Simply mention pollen, and all those unfortunate enough to have suffered from 'hay fever', the common term for a collection of symptoms linked to spring allergies, will by instinct suffer from a tingling in their throat, itchy eyes and a runny nose. And yet they would probably be surprised to learn that pollen can become their best ally.

In point of fact, there are two sorts of pollen. Pollens that are wind-borne, in so-called anemophilic pollination, are those principally responsible for the triggering of allergic reactions by the immune system: they are allergens.

By contrast, pollens that are collected by bees or other insects, in what is called entomophilous fertilization, are hypoallergenic. The regulatory role they play on the immune system has been demonstrated on several occasions. By acting as a form of vaccine, they allow desensitising to take place and this results in the progressive disappearance of allergic symptoms (rhinitis, asthma). With the help of other products from the hive, in particular certain bee-venom extracts which are also very efficient and seldom used for desensitising, apitherapy is remarkably high performing in the fight against allergies.

Many projects, carried out at various universities, have confirmed

9. A PHARMACOPEIA DIRECT FROM THE HIVE

the validity of these protocols, which have been devised by scientists who were passionate about apiculture and who have understood the importance of working from the fundamental notion of re-establishing our relationship with nature.

Royal jelly.

Royal jelly is secreted by the pharyngeal glands of young bees, otherwise known as nurse bees. It is used to feed all eggs from the first to the third day, then those larvae destined to become queens, and the queen herself for the whole of her life.

Thanks to this exceptional foodstuff, the queen is able to lay daily a number of eggs equivalent to that of her own body weight – 1,500 eggs per day on average – and to live for three to five years, whereas the life expectancy of a worker bee does not exceed six weeks during the active season.

Harvesting this substance demands specific technical know-how and even then the quantities produced are tiny, which explains its high price. For a few years now it has been possible to purchase frozen royal jelly from China, at a price as low as to mirror its quality.

Composition of royal jelly:-

Water: between 64% and 66%
Carbohydrates: between 12% and 16%, fructose and glucose in equal parts.
Lipids: between 4% and 6%
Proteins: between 12% and 18%, ie in lesser quantities than in pollen, but still containing the eight essential amino-acids

Vitamins, in particular all vitamins from the B group except for B12 which is only present at trace levels. Royal jelly is the natural substance richest in vitamin B5, pantothenate, which is the quintessential anti-stress vitamin and which has an anti-fatigue action and promotes longevity.

Minerals and trace elements.

Around 3% of various other substances, some of which have not yet been fully identified, including acetylcholin and some antibacterial agents.

*

Royal jelly has often been described as a miracle remedy capable of curing all illnesses. This is probably a little bit over-enthusiastic. However, it is the case that its properties make it highly recommended in the treatment of a number of complaints, or simply as a preventative or for general fitness.

Royal jelly has a crucial influence on the intracellular metabolism, the cardio-vascular system, the digestive system, the immune system, the endocrine system, the nervous system and the mind. More generally, it can be said that it has stimulant, fortifying and euphoriant effects, and that it is a useful aid against problems due to ageing, be it at organ or skin level, or even in respect of intellectual faculties thanks to its ability to appreciably increase oxygen flow to the brain.

Propolis.

Whereas everybody is capable of referring to honey, royal jelly, wax or pollen, not many people know about propolis, least of all its origin and properties.

The name pro-polis, which is of Greek origin, means "before the city"; an impregnable battlement, therefore. Some even refer to it as the hive's armoury, or as a veritable natural 'antibiotic'.

When a predator, such as a field mouse or a lizard for instance, goes into a hive to gorge on honey, logically it is killed by the guard bees. But as the insects don't have the strength to drag it outside, they wrap the corpse with a layer of propolis; this mummifies it and prevents decomposition. It is likely that ancient Egyptians had observed this phenomenon before they refined their embalmment processes, which confirms the antifungal properties of propolis.

What could be more logical? In a confined space occupied by tens of thousands of insects who come and go and bustle restlessly at temperatures between 35° and 38° with a relative humidity of 70%, and with its high sugar content, the hive ought to be an absolute culture broth. Yet, it is generally a model of hygiene, thanks mostly to the presence of propolis.

9. A PHARMACOPEIA DIRECT FROM THE HIVE

This exceptional substance comes from the thin resin layer which covers buds, that is to say the envelope with which trees protect their most precious assets: their progeny, their future.

In the first days of spring and autumn bees harvest propolis from birch trees, alders, horse chestnuts, oaks, poplars, willows and the bark of spruce trees. They use their mandibles to chop it into small fragments that can then be transported, like pollen, in baskets situated on the bees' hind legs.

Bees then mix the propolis with saliva secretions and variable proportions of beeswax in order to obtain a sort of putty which they use to plug any holes or cracks and to ensure an airtight environment within the hive, but above all enabling permanent disinfection to take place. Besides, the area in front of the hive entrance is coated with propolis, forming a footbath to enable foragers' feet to be cleaned upon return.

*

It is absolutely essential that the harvesting of this substance should be strictly controlled. The traditional method, which consisted in scraping the frames, is being gradually discarded as it used to bring in too many impurities. Nowadays, conscientious beekeepers have to work with either a mesh or a layer of gauze, a process which preserves the quality of the propolis.

Propolis is a mixture of resins and balsams issued from plants (55%), vegetable wax (30%), essential oils (5% to 10%), pollen (5%) and various organic and mineral substances (5%); it comprises 150 different elements and is an endless source of anti-oxidants (principally flavonoid compounds in our part of the world), as well as phenolic and aromatic components, not to mention a wide range of trace elements.

In order to achieve a standardisation in manufacture according to therapeutic requirements and also to render propolis 100% bio-assimilable, a re-concentrating technique has been developed and this makes it possible to obtain a product which is 10 to 20 times more potent than raw propolis.

*

However, as is the case with honey and pollen, it is not really possible to speak about simply 'propolis' since there are several varieties all with different plant origins and with specific effects. It has taken years of laboratory studies and field studies to develop a procedure that makes it possible to exploit the essential powerful elements that all types of propolis offer. To date there are 11 listed types, all of them the subjects of various scientific papers which demonstrate their distinct physical and chemical properties. Unfortunately, few are commercialized in sufficient quantities to be used in the pharmaceutical industry. There are at the moment only three types of propolis widely available.

In order to facilitate classification, a colour-coding system is used.

Red propolis, whose specific antiviral properties have been mostly studied in the Americas and Cuba.

Brown propolis, whose specific antibacterial properties have been studied mainly in Europe.

Green propolis, whose specific anti-cancer properties have been principally studied in Japan.

Others, such as black propolis and yellow propolis, are still under study.

Clearly, as always in the domain of natural medicine, each main specific tendency has to be determined, but it is obvious that nothing in nature is ever that simple. There is a cross-over of the different properties while each type of propolis retains its singularity.

Clinical studies carried out by "official" medicine would have the power to establish, clearly and without dispute, the extraordinary therapeutic powers of this substance, which could advantageously replace a number of drugs and some of the often inefficacious treatments, in particular in the field of hospital-acquired infections, one of public health's gravest problems nowadays. As always though, it is only a question of open-mindedness.

ENT disorders.

The use of antibiotics for the treatment of infections in the upper respiratory tract is still extremely frequent today. The necessity of this is, however, strongly called into question. In point of fact, a detailed analysis dating back to 2007 has, following a detailed comparative study of a large collection of data, put forward the case that prescribing antibiotics for this kind of infection, which is still the most common cause of visits to the doctor, is ineffective in the majority of cases, and that it can contribute to the increase in incidences of resistant strains.

9. A PHARMACOPEIA DIRECT FROM THE HIVE

In this type of condition, the tests that help distinguish between viral and bacterial infections are unfortunately rarely used by the medical profession, and in the absence of clinical criteria it is all the more difficult to reach a diagnosis. Generally, the practitioner's attitude follows two main directions: either he prescribes a broad-spectrum antibiotic in order to cover all of the most likely causes, or he decides to treat the symptoms. Both approaches are but approximate solutions. It must be noted that the prescribing of antibiotics also seems to occur in response to patients' own expectations

However, this 2007 study demonstrates that antibiotics do not appear to be beneficial in the case of ENT infections, since they do not bring about any improvements in the patient's condition.

This widespread recognition, along with an evolution in attitudes, goes a long way to encourage practitioners as well as patients to turn to alternative treatments, using products from natural medicine.

The surprising properties of some of these natural substances in the treatment of viral or bacterial respiratory infections have been confirmed by a large number of studies over the last few years. One of the most analysed of these substances happens to be propolis. Its properties have been widely evidenced in scientific literature. Its action appears to be both preventative and therapeutic, and it is particularly well adapted to the treatment of upper respiratory tract infections.

As a matter of fact, the beneficial effects of propolis on ENT illnesses have been demonstrated on acute ear inflammations and rhinitis. More recently, a study carried out on 94 patients has revealed a decrease in the number of cases of nasopharyngitis amongst the subjects treated with propolis when compared with a control group who had received no treatment at all. A study carried out in 2000 has also been able to demonstrate here the antimicrobial action of propolis on Streptococcus pyogenes, which is one of the main agents responsible for pharyngitis and sore throats in children.

Finally, the Canadian Ministry for Health, acting as a precursor to the official recognition of natural health remedies, has just published a monograph which recognizes the therapeutic effects of propolis on throat infections and deals with their treatment and relief. Moreover, Canada Health underlines the mucolytic properties of this substance from the hive.

A clinical study carried out in 2004 among 430 patients has proved that the effects of propolis on ENT disorders appears to be reinforced when used in conjunction with vitamin C. The authors also suggest that the decrease in local concentration of both viruses and bacteria in the nasopharynx can be attributed to the anti-inflammatory and decongestant properties found in a product combining propolis with vitamin C. Therefore it appears that there is a strengthening in effects, that is to say a synergy, between these two substances.

All this also confirms the works of Doctor Teresa Giral Rivera's team in Cuba; since 1995 they have been highlighting the particularly strong properties of Cuban red propolis when applied to viral infections in the upper respiratory tract, as well as on type A and B 'flu viruses. The same goes for the work that we have carried out for four years within hospitals on the same island, acting jointly for the Apitherapy Commission and the Finlay Institute. The main assets of propolis as evidenced in these studies remain its anti-inflammatory, antiviral and mucolytic properties. Faced with ENT diseases, which can have multiple origins, propolis whether associated with essential oils or not, appears to offer a particularly well-suited alternative treatment. Furthermore, to this day this substance has shown no, or very few, known side effects, and almost no cases of allergies have been listed.

Red propolis and herpes.

The herpes virus inhabits 85% of the European human population, and we will have to get used to living with it. 15% of these microbes are already resistant to classic antiviral treatments. Some people have very regular eruptions not only on the corners of the lips but also on external parts of their genitalia. These are the most frequent symptoms.

Red propolis, which has been selected for its specific antiviral, anti-inflammatory and wound-healing properties, makes for good tissue regeneration. It is the go-to product for this type of pathology. Complementary studies have demonstrated that this particular propolis brings about a marked decrease in recurrence, which is otherwise very frequent in this type of condition.

This substance is harvested by honeybees on mangroves. This is what appears to give it its coloration, but most of all its biochemical specificity, hence its therapeutic specificity. It is therefore one of the

9. A PHARMACOPEIA DIRECT FROM THE HIVE

most studied propolis in the world. Its composition makes it particularly active against the most resistant of viruses. Modern techniques enable us to highlight some types of propolis whose particular therapeutic properties have been recognized. Green medicine is derived from traditional medicine but it has to acquire its power and credibility through biochemical modernity which has been validated by universities.

In order to fight herpes for the long term and in an even more radical manner, an extract of red propolis combined with essential oils – melaleuca quinquenervia cineolifera and ocimum basilicum var. Basilicum – will have exceptional antiseptic and antiviral properties. The combined action of phenolic acids and flavonoids contained in this propolis with the chemo-types from the chosen aromatic plants is quite remarkable. This combination has been successfully tested on many hospital cases.

Once it had successfully gone through all the pre-clinical and clinical phases, this preparation was listed as a natural medicine against herpes simplex 1 (lips) and 2 (genitals) as well as against herpes zoster (shingles) in Cuba in 2005.

Green propolis and cancer.

A large number of publications have shown that propolis from Brazil, and more precisely from the tree "baccharis dracunculifolia", also known as alecrim-do-campo or field rosemary, can favourably be used in conjunction with chemotherapies and that it combats the development of cancer cells through various active mechanisms.

The concentrated flavonoids contained in green propolis have very efficacious anti-oxidizing powers. Propolis extract shows the capture of free radicals. The point being, cell oxidization is one of the most frequent factors in cancer cases.

Ethanolic extracts from green propolis have shown both cytotoxic and cytostatic effects in vitro against ovarian cancerous tumours and sarcoma tumours in rats. Phenethyl ester of caffeic acid shows a cytotoxic action in cultures of tumour cells, both human and animal: breast carcinoma, melanoma, colon cancer and kidney cancer. Another substance isolated from green propolis, artepillin C, shows a cytotoxic effect in vitro against humain gastric carcinoma cells, lung carcinoma cells and also on colon cancer cells from rats.

Propolis is also capable of stimulating immune responses in rats. More recently, Japanese researchers have demonstrated the relation between propolis extract and the activation of macrophages linked to immune functions in humans.

Propolis is more efficacious than its components. Some components, although known for their anti-cancerous activity, are less efficient in delaying the development of metastases when they are administered on their own than when propolis is given directly to mice. For comparison, untreated mice developed an average of 62 metastases. When caffeic acid injections are added, the figure falls to 43, whereas with propolis it is 22. Researchers have therefore drawn the conclusion that there is a synergy between the various components, which optimizes their effect. (It is worth noting that when the treatments have been applied as a preventative measure, ie before the onset of cancer, results have been even better.)

Two types of study have confirmed that green propolis reinforces the action of chemotherapy. The first instance has been demonstrated by a team in Zagreb. First of all, they noticed that propolis was more efficient than the product commonly used alongside chemotherapy: Epirubicin. Against the average 62 metastases that occur in untreated mice, chemotherapy can reduce the numbers to an average of 28, and propolis to 15! There is no question of replacing the former by the latter however because in the second instance Croatian researchers have shown that if you administer both chemotherapy and propolis the number of metastases now falls to 4!

The second, a Japanese study, has reached equivalent results in respect of the volume of tumours. When associated with either mitomycin or 5-FU, two cancer treatment drugs, propolis stops the growth of tumours after three weeks, whereas chemotherapies only manage to slow it down.

The side effects of chemotherapy are well documented. Amongst others, the lowering of blood counts, especially a significant loss of white and red cells, often compromises the chances of continuing with the treatment. Once again, if propolis is associated with the chemotherapy treatment, surprising results are achieved. White corpuscles are still reduced in numbers, but by half the amounts. Red corpuscle numbers are restored to near normal levels after 35 days' treatment.

9. A PHARMACOPEIA DIRECT FROM THE HIVE

So, here are six good reasons which prove that, when associated with classic treatments, green propolis brings about undeniable added value.

However, research goes even further.

In the course of the last thirty years, our understanding of cancer has been fundamentally altered by the discovery of the genes which are responsible for the development of this illness. Today, researchers are examining the transducers for these genes, and more specifically an enzyme called PAK1, which may be responsible for the molecular activation that leads to cell division, the invasion of the body by the tumour, the survival of cancerous cells and the development of blood vessels within the tumour.

Current research is therefore working on the preparation of drugs designed to block the activity of PAK1 They would reduce the mitosis (cell division) of cancer cells at source, but also the formation of metastases, reduce angiogenisis (the development of new blood vessels by budding from existing vessels), and re-establish apoptosis, that is to say the pre-programmed cell death which has ceased occurring among cancer cells.

Numerous studies have proved that Ser/Thrkinase PAK1, to give it its full scientific name, is an essential transducer in more than 70% of cancers, among which those of the upper respiratory tract, prostate, and neurofibromatosis.

These tumours, which are highly dependent on the presence of this kinase for their growth, are therefore called "PAK1-dependent".

Given that the development of synthetic "PAK1 blocking" drugs will take many years, research is turning to natural products which would offer the same powers, in the hope that patients will benefit sooner from this new therapeutic approach. Amongst these natural products, one of the most promising seems to be green propolis from Brazil, which is rich in Artepillin C, an excellent "PAK1 blocker".

*

In traditional medicine, it is well known that propolis possesses a large spectrum of therapeutic properties, amongst which are anti-hepatotoxic, anti-inflammatory and anti-oxidant actions. Its anti-cancerous activity, however, is without doubt its most promising medicinal property, and the one that is most studied the world over. Green propolis from Brazil is the only type to contain 6% to 8% Artepillin C.

Scientific publications mention several studies relating to the anti-cancerous properties of the active ingredient in green propolis, as well as its biochemical modus operandi. In 2005, a team of Japanese researchers highlighted the anti-proliferative action of ARC on cancer cells of the human colon. The following year, the same researchers published the review of a study based on mice given propolis by mouth. In this, they illustrate the properties of both ARC and propolis, which have both been absorbed well. These two substances have triggered an anti-oxidant reaction in the body by means of the production of detoxifying enzymes which neutralize the ravages inflicted by oxidizing free radicals; this reaction has been reinforced by the presence in propolis of many flavonoids.

According to many authors, oxidizing damage can lead to mutations which in turn lead to the emergence of cancerous lesions. However, the inhibiting action of ARC on colon lesion in mice appears to be very efficacious.

According to a study carried out in 2007, this action would appear to be accompanied by anti-angiogenesis properties. Indeed, researchers have observed a significant reduction in numbers in the emergence of new blood vessels within tumours in mice treated with propolis administered by mouth.

Finally, a study published in 2009 clearly demonstrated that ARC and green propolis block the PAK1 signal selectively. Their important therapeutic effects on the growth of neuro-fibromatous tumours have also been evidenced both in vitro and in vivo.

As their research progresses, scientists appear to be discovering Artepillin C' increasing powers. More than 70% of cancers being "PAK1-dependent" and Artepillin C seems to be a very efficient "PAK1 blocker".

It is therefore anticipated that Green propolis from Brazil, which is very rich in Artepillin C, will offer a complementary natural remedy against cancer. It is one of the rare substances studied as potential complements to classic chemotherapies, and it has demonstrated that its association with chemotherapy was far more efficacious than hospital treatments on their own. The "PAK1 blocker" is readily absorbed by

9. A PHARMACOPEIA DIRECT FROM THE HIVE

the body. It seems easy to administer orally, and there is a possibility that a daily dose could have inhibiting powers against certain types of cancer.

The Japanese, who are simultaneously at the forefront of modernity and rooted in tradition, routinely use concentrated green propolis tincture as a preventative treatment. This use represents a market worth more than one billion dollars a year!

Venom.

Only female bees are equipped with a stinging mechanism, which consists of two juxtaposed stingers. The males, called drones, don't sting. Neither do they do any work. Their only task is to fertilize the queen. They are idlers and once they have become redundant in the autumn they are killed or chased out of the hive.

Bee venom is secreted from both acid and base glands. It is a clear liquid, with a strong characteristic smell. The type of venom produced by the queen is only used to despatch her rivals; it acts immediately and is less concentrated than that of a worker bee, whose venom evolves during her lifetime and varies according to the seasons and also apparently according to her nutrition.

The bee only uses her stinger in order to defend her nest and her family. She has to be jostled or disturbed before she decides to sting. She never carries out unprovoked attacks and never stings without good reason.

Composition of bee venom:-

Water: around 85%

Volatile components: 2% to 3%. Venom contains numerous essences which are very important from a curative point of view. This is one of the reasons why the use of stings from live bees is preferable rather than reconstituted venom, which will have lost most of its essential oils.

The following are found in the remaining 12% or so:-

13% to 15% enzymes, in particular phospholipase A2, but also esterases, phospholipase B, phosphatises and hyaluronidase.

55% to 60% proteins and peptides, in particular mellitin, but also the peptide responsible for the granulation of mastocytes (MCD peptide), apamine, minomine, cardiopeptide, histamine and dopamine.

25% to 30% non-animate components; phospholipids, simple sugars, glucose and fructose, vanillymandelic acid and oligosaccharides.

*

As is the case with many "poisons" in nature, rational use of bee venom enables us to obtain therapeutic solutions of a high order.

Paracelse, a Swiss doctor and alchemist from the sixteenth century, said it clearly: "Any substance can be both venom and medicine; it all depends on the dose that is administered."

Other than in cases of known allergies, the phobia about "killer bees" is unfounded. It takes more than a thousand stings to kill an adult. When we administer twenty to forty stings per session, we are therefore very far from giving a fatal dose, and well below the danger zone.

The same cannot be said about chemical drugs, whose excessive and thoughtless use leads to several hundred deaths every year in France alone. And this happens without any voices being raised.

Bee Venom Therapy is ancient. In the fourth century BC, Hippocrates already referred to it, and it is said that both Charlemagne and Ivan the Terrible resorted to it against their bouts of gout.

Today, results are clear and the sixty thousand people who get themselves treated by this process in the United States can bear witness as to its efficacy. Bee venom acts principally on rheumatism, auto-immune disorders, some pressure sores and skin cancers.

Yet, the medical world still refuses to use it, and the big labs do not like it when we remind people of bee venom's excellent vasodilatator properties. Could this have anything to do with the gigantic market for this type of drug that exists in our western society?

Wax.

Beeswax is secreted by the worker bees' wax glands, from day 11 of

9. A PHARMACOPEIA DIRECT FROM THE HIVE

their lives until they start flying out of the hive a week later. The bee kneads the wax in her mouth and each little wax blob is deposited alongside the previous one in perfect alignment in order to construct cells arranged in a honeycomb constructed vertically, starting at the top.

The cells are hexagonal in shape and their strength, regularity and beauty means that bees are the best architects in nature. Furthermore, since bees are thrifty – and since wax production is costly in terms of energy consumption – this chosen geometrical shape enables the structure to be the strongest possible whilst using the fewest materials.

*

The composition of wax is very complex. Each of the main constituents is itself a combination of other, simpler elements. They include:-

Esters from fatty acids and alcohols: 70%
Free acids: 14%
Hydrocarbons: 12%
Free alcohols: 1.2%
Lactones: 0.5%
Water and other substances: 2%

During the course of history, wax has been mostly used as an excipient in many preparations, in particular suppositories and pessaries. When mixed with cocoa butter at a rate of 6.05%, its melting point is exactly 37°C. It has enabled the manufacture of ointments, cerates, and pomades.

Applied externally, it has been used for cicatrising, or in poultices for the treatment of rheumatism.

Taken internally in the form of flakes encased within capsules, it has a beneficial effect on some types of diarrhoea or on constipation. Wax also has anti-inflammatory properties.

Nowadays it is mostly used in cosmetics.

Essential oils.

Four thousand years before Jesus Christ, in China, India, Persia, Egypt, then in Greece and under the Roman Empire, aromatic plants were already used as medicines. Sacred texts refer to this many a time.

An essential oil is obtained through the distillation of an aromatic plant using water vapour. It is not to be confused with essences, which are obtained by a simple extraction process, in particular in the case of citrus fruit.

Despite its name, an essential oil does not contain any fats. The name comes from the fact that due to its density it rises to the surface of water.

*

Essential oils are complex substances, being arrangements of various aromatic molecules, each with its own particular properties. Determining which vegetal species the essential oil has been extracted from is not sufficient to determine its therapeutic value. It is necessary to define the essential oil by its main chemical component: this notion is that of a chemotype, or chemical race.

For instance, the species thymus vulgaris, despite its unvarying appearance – same leaves, same flowers, same pollen grains, and same genome – will synthesize different main components according to its natural habitat, or biotope. Therefore different chemotypes of thymus vulgaris will give their essential oils very distinct therapeutic values:-

thymus vulgaris geranioliferum
thymus vulgaris linaloliferum
thymus vulgaris paracymeniferum
thymus vulgaris thujanoliferum
thymus vulgaris thymoliferum

A rigorous classification of these chemical traces will avoid errors in usage and allows for appropriate medical use. There are twelve biochemical component families. The specific therapeutic action of each of these essential oils is defined very precisely by the value, quality and percentage of these components.

*

Today there are more than 250 essential oils in common use. Honey is the ideal vessel for their penetration and for their uptake by the body. Such a mixture, within which each will multiply the properties

9. A PHARMACOPEIA DIRECT FROM THE HIVE

of the others ad infinitum, enables us to build up a non-exhaustive pharmacopeia: aroma-honeys.

10. Medicine from the Honeybees

Apitherapy is a global health concept which, since its components are produced by Mother Nature, makes for the most harmonious of preventative and curative medicines. The use of natural products leads to the acceptance of impermanence, the very principle of life according to the Dalai Lama.

*

In chemistry as in synthetic drug production, the active materials are molecules which are defined and invariable, which leads to the growth of, among others, resistant bacteria that have a stupendous ability to adapt.

One of green medicine's great strengths is that, despite the products' temporal variations, their action remains unchanged. Faced with this, bacteria and viruses are virtually unable to adapt. This medicine is therefore more efficient, both at the time of use and for the future.

*

Illness is the result of an aggression against our body, either from outside – via viruses or bacteria - or internally – generated consciously or unconsciously by the individuals themselves when under stress. More often than not, there exists a subtle and complex mix between the "agent" and the "terrain".

Such aggression overpowers our natural immunological defences, leading to the onset of a disease that will last for a shorter or longer period of time. Sometimes the illness takes hold and leads the body into a state I would call chronic "pathological equilibrium".

Classical medicine will firstly attempt to identify the external aggressive agent and to deploy targeted means to fight it vigorously. In accordance with standard practice, diagnosis is simplified by resorting to "broad spectrum" therapeutic actions which are directed against a whole range of potential infectious agents.

This approach, although its results are generally uncontested, is not without unwanted side effects. It results in serious pollution of the body, sometimes even leading to iatrogenic conditions which can on occasion prove fatal.

In all cases, patients are exhausted by the ordeal, as much from the illness itself as from the shock treatments that have been dispensed. Patients' immune defences, which have been taken over by chemicals, are reduced in the extreme. This is the phenomenon called immunodeficiency, described in leaflets that hardly anybody reads and which leaves the door wide open to new aggressions and to relapse.

Apitherapy on the contrary is contained within a process of natural medicine which consists in fighting the aggressor whilst boosting the immune system.

One of the basic principles is to overthrow the state of "pathological equilibrium" by provoking a crisis. This destabilization can be accompanied by a temporary worsening of symptoms, which leads to a belief that there has been a sudden degradation, whereas it is in fact the first step on the road to recovery. It corresponds to the time it takes the body to gets its defence systems back to "fighting fit" status.

The treatment will help the body along by providing it with the substances necessary for the task, even directly supplying elements that will fight directly against the external agent where necessary, or else bringing about protocols for detoxification if necessary.

*

Apitherapy can offer practitioners a number of tools which form a veritable armoury with which to respond. In many cases, even in severe illnesses, experience has shown us that they are very successful.

Some circumstances can call for the build up of a synergy between apitherapy and other appropriate medical protocols. The practitioner will always need to use his or her critical thinking in order to offer patients the most appropriate solution, whilst always bearing in mind the fundamental principle of medicine, as enunciated by Hippocrates:

10. MEDICINE FROM THE HONEYBEES

"First of all, do no harm."

Notes.

You will find below a list of the various diseases that products from the hive are likely to treat.

If these products have the power to cure, they can also, through regular treatment, prevent diseases as far as prevention is possible.

We need to bear in mind the simple but perennial principle that "prevention is better than cure."

*

The lives we lead today demand from our bodies a formidable and constant capacity to adapt, all the more since our only hope to cleanse them is via the air we breathe. Nutrition now plays a crucial role and must be, as much as a way to feed ourselves, a means to guard against aggressions.

We must therefore follow a few common sense principles in our behaviour in order to enable us to face difficult situations with the minimum of damage.

(1) Our health's four great enemies are alcohol, tobacco, fats and rapid sugars. These are responsible for an infinite number of diseases (particularly in view of the fact that their consumption is often associated), and must be banished without hesitation. Red wine does not need to be included in this list, provided that it is consumed in moderation, to a rate of six to ten glasses a week, and it must still be possible to party where special circumstances occur! From time to time, excesses are good for the soul and for health.

(2) Cereals, vegetables and fruit, a variety of them in all their forms, must constitute the lion's share of our nutrition: it is at last recognized that vegetable proteins, which have for a long time been considered as negligible, can indeed replace animal proteins.

(3) These are simple truths that we are all aware of, even if we don't apply them. What is less well known however is that dairy products, contrary to their reputation, are not good for our health. Milk, even

skimmed milk, is too rich in fats and proteins. Paradoxically, in order to eliminate these, the body has to consume the calcium that milk was supposed to be providing in the first place. One of these proteins, casein, sticks to the walls of the entire digestive system and provokes a putrid fermentation which is at the source of many an inflammation.

These are only the "natural" drawbacks of milk, which has forever been presented to us as an ideal foodstuff. If you add to it two substances with which cows are regularly injected: antibiotics to fight infections and growth hormones (carcinogenic) to increase productivity, you will understand why an American biologist, Robert Cohen, created a scandal in the United States with his book: Milk, the deadly poison.

It is therefore obvious that in order to ensure maximum efficacy each of the recommended treatments must be accompanied by a total removal of dairy products, including cheese, from the diet.

10. MEDICINE FROM THE HONEYBEES

11. Therapeutic Usage of Products from the Hive

Advice.

All the products you purchase must always be from an organic source, which is a sine qua non guarantee of quality. Essential oils must be 'chemotyped' (biochemically defined).

The preparation of a curative aroma-honey to be taken orally follows the following formula: 3g to 5g of essential oils to each 100g honey. Given that a gramme contains roughly 25 drops, you can prepare the mixture, stirring it for a good five minutes, using the easy-to-remember formula 100 drops of essential oils to 100g honey.

If several essential oils are included in the aroma-honey, simply divide 100 drops by the number of essential oils.

For external applications, the ratio has to be brought down to 25 drops of essential oils to 100g honey.

The usual dosage is as follows:-

Three teaspoons per day for ten days for acute conditions
One tablespoon twice a day, for up to a month, for chronic conditions

Doses are to be taken before meals, placing the aroma-honey under the tongue where it is to be kept for several minutes until completely dissolved in saliva. The tongue is one of the parts of the body that is richest in blood capillaries, which ensures an instant and optimal diffusion, since it by-passes the filter that is the liver.

*

Propo-honey is prepared as follows: 10g of original propolis tincture, at a 25% concentration, for each 100g of honey whenever it is administered orally. The dosage is identical to that for aroma-honeys.

If applied externally, the rate falls to 2g of original tincture per

100g honey.

*

Whenever pollen is recommended, ideally fresh pollen should be taken. If you are unable to procure this, then choose dry pollen. The usual dosage is as follows:- one teaspoon twice a day, taken before meals.

As far as propolis is concerned, opt for capsules (and take 4 to 6 per day).

*

Products from the hive do not have any toxic side effects. A few rare cases of allergies have been recorded.

*

There is no negative interaction between the different products, and they can be taken together, separately, or as a complement to chemical treatments.

All the above dosages are for adults weighing between 45kg and 100kgs.

11. THERAPEUTIC USAGE OF PRODUCTS FROM THE HIVE

ALPHABETICAL LISTING OF AILMENTS

Acne.
Propo-aroma-honey: thyme honey + Alcoholic tincture of propolis + essential oil of thymus vulgaris (linalool) • Propolis cleansing cream.

Aerophagia.
Pollen • Propolis • Aroma-honey: lemon blossom honey + essential oils of citrus reticulate and ocimum basilicum basilicum.
OR: • Aroma-honey: wild thyme honey + essential oils of pimpinella anisum and carum carvi.

Ageing.
Royal jelly • Mountain multi-flower honey • Pollen.

Allergies.
Bee bread • Apipuncture - micro-stinging administered by a specialist practitioner • Aroma-honey: rosemary honey + essential oils of helichrysum italicum, citrus limonum (zest), rosmarinus officinalis (1.8 cineol).
OR: • Aroma-honey: mountain multi-floral honey + essential oils of helichrysum italicum, chamaemelum nobile and citrus limonum (zest).

Amebiasis.
Propolis • Aroma-honey: lavender honey + essential oils of cymbopogon citratus, origanum compactum, thymus vulgaris (linalool) and satureja montana.

Amenorrhea.
Royal jelly • Aroma-honey: heather honey + essential oils of cupressus

sempervirens and salvia officinalis.

Anaemia.
Pollen • Royal jelly • Heather honey or Miel de Sapin1(*) or rosemary honey.

Anxiety.
Pollen from orange blossom • Lime blossom honey • Aroma-honey: orange blossom honey + essential oil of citrus aurantium petitgrain/bergamot or citrus aurantium neroli/bigarade or citrus aurantium petit grain/mandarin.

Aphonia.
Lavender honey • Thyme honey • Miel de sapin* • Propo-honey with above honeys.

Arteriosclerosis.
Pollen • Rosemary honey, hawthorn honey • Propo-honey with rosemary honey • Aroma-honey: rosemary honey + essential oils of cupressus sempervirens, citrus reticulata, cedrus atlantica and apium graveolens.

Arteritis.
Alcoholic tincture of propolis • Aroma-honey: heather honey or sweet-chestnut honey + essential oils from Artemisia dracunculus, rosmarinus officinalis (verbenon), helichrisum italicum and citrus limonum (zest)

Arthritis.
Bee venom: in ointment, in cream, through stinging by a specialist practitioner • Propolis • Pollen • Aroma-honey: rosemary honey + essential oils of eucalyptus citriodora, laurus nobilis, origanum marjorana and junuperus communis communis.

Asthenia (Weakness).
Pollen • Royal jelly • Bee bread • Mountain multi-floral honey + royal

jelly.

Asthma.

Propolis • Apipuncture - micro-stinging administered by a specialist practitioner • Desensitization by pollen • Miel de Sapin* • Aroma-honey: eucalyptus honey + essential oils of eucalyptus globulus, eucalyptus radiate and rosemary (1.8 cineol) • Aroma-honey: Miel de Sapin* + essential oils of pinus sylvestris and artemisia draconculus.

Blood Acidity.

Pollen.

Blood Acetone.

Pollen • Propolis • Sage honey.

Bloating.

Pollen • Propolis • Aroma-honey: rosemary honey + essential oils of rosmarinus officinalis (verbenon) + essential oil of foeniculum vulgare dulce (common fennel).

Boils (External Treatment).

Thyme propo-honey • Aroma-honey: thyme honey + essential oil of thymus (geraniol) • + essential oil of melaleuca alternifolia.

Breast Feeding.

Royal jelly • Fresh pollen • Mountain multi-floral honey.

Bronchitis.

Propolis • Propolis tincture • Aroma-honey: eucalyptus or lavender or Miel de Sapin* + essential oil of eucalyptus radiate + essential oil of eucalyptus globules + essential oil of rosmarinus officinalis (1.8 cineol).

Bulimia.

Pollen • Bee bread • Aroma-honey: multi-floral mountain honey + essential oil of origanum majorana + essential oil of thymus vulgaris (linalool) + essential oil of anethum graveolens + essential oil of mentha citrate.

Burns.
Cool down by running the burnt area under fresh water for a few minutes • Multi-floral mountain honey, lavender honey, sweet chestnut honey, thyme honey. All the above must have been standardized for therapeutic use • Propo-aroma-honey: 1% propolis tincture at a 50% concentration.

Cancer.
This is in addition to medical treatment.
Green propolis • Pollen • Aroma-honey: thyme or sweet chestnut honey + essential oil of ravensara aromatic + essential oil of melaleuca quinquinerva + essential oil of laurus nobilis.

Cancerous Tumours.
In addition to medical treatment:
Propolis • Bee bread • Aroma-honey: mountain multi-flower honey + essential oil of daucus carota + essential oil of laurus nobilis + essential oil of ravensara aromatica + essential oil of juniperus communis (berries).

Candida Vaginitis.
Pessaries made up of alcoholic propolis tincture + essential oil of origanum majorana + essential oil of melaleuca alternifolia.

Chapping.
Local treatment with beeswax + propolis tincture. Local application of lavender or mountain wildflower honey.

Chilblains.
Lavender honey applied in a poultice • Lavender propo-honey applied in a poultice.

Cholesterol.
Propolis • Pollen • Aroma-honey: rosemary or thyme honey + essential oil of helichrisum italicum + essential oil of rosmarinus officinalis (verbenon acetate) + essential oil of laurus nobilis.

Cirrhosis.
Propolis • Pollen • Aroma-honey: rosemary or thyme honey + essential oil of mentha piperata + essential oil of daucus carota.

Cold.
Royal jelly • Miel de Sapin* honey • Propolis • Propolis tincture.

Colibacillocis.
Propolis • Aroma-honey: heather or thyme honey + essential oil of melaleuca alternifolia + essential oil of thymus vulgaris (linalool) + essential oil of satureja montana.

Colic.
Pollen • Propolis • Thyme honey.

Colitis.
Pollen • Propolis • Aroma-honey: multi-floral mountain honey + essential oil of melaleuca alternifolia + essential oil of rosmarinus officinalis (verbenon).

Common Cold.
Propolis • Eucalyptus honey • Aroma-honey: eucalyptus honey + essential oil of eucalyptus globulus + essential oil of rosmarinus (1.8 cineol) + essential oil of inula graveolens.

Constipation.
Pollen • Beeswax flakes taken either by spoon or in capsules • Acacia honey.

Corysa.
Propolis • Aroma-honey: thyme honey + essential oil of thyme (linalool) + essential oil of rosmarinus officinalis (cineol 1.8) + essential oil of ocimum basilicum basilicum.

Coughing.
Mountain multi-flower honey, lavender honey, Miel de Sapin* honey or eucalyptus honey • Alcoholic tincture of propolis • Propo-honey made

from the above-mentioned honeys • Aroma-honey: eucalyptus honey + essential oil of eucalyptus radiata + essential oil of eucalyptus smitii.

Cracked Skin.
Aroma-honey: lemon blossom honey + essential oil of citrus lemon • Propolis cream • Lavender honey applied in poultices.

Cystitis.
Propolis • Aroma-honey: lavender or thyme or heather honey + essential oil of mentha piperata + essential oil of satureja montana + essential oil of salvia officinalis.

Diabetes.
Aroma-honey: acacia honey, essential oil of pelargonium graveolens + essential oil of anethum graveolens + essential oil of eucalyptus citriodora + essential oil of juniperus communis (berries) • Pollen • Bee bread • Propolis.

Diarrhoea.
Pollen • Propolis • Bee bread • Aroma-honey: thyme honey + essential oil of origanum majorana + essential oil of officinal rosmarinus (verbenon) or Aroma-honey: thyme honey + essential oil of mentha piperata.

Decalcification and Demineralization.
Propolis • Bee bread • Buckwheat honey.

Dermatitis.
Thyme honey • Propo-honey • Aroma-honey: lavender honey, essential oil of angustifolia (vera) + essential oil of thymus vulgaris (linalol).

Dysentery.
Pollen • Propolis • Bee bread • Aroma-honey: thyme honey + essential oil of mentha piperata.

Dyspepsia (Digestion Problems).
Rosemary honey or thyme/wild thyme honey, or lemon blossom honey

• Pollen • Propolis • Aroma-honey: orange blossom honey + essential oil of citrus aurantium (peel).

Ear Infection.
Propolis tincture (local application) • Propolis • Aroma-honey: thyme honey + essential oil of thymus vulgaris (linalool) + essential oil of thymus vulgaris (thujanol) + essential oil of eucalyptus radiata used in local application (total essential oil concentration 1%) as well as orally.

Eczema.
Lavender honey applied directly to the skin • Propo-honey applied directly to the skin • Aroma-honey: lavender honey + essential oil of lavandula angustifolia (vera) applied directly to the skin • Aroma-honey: rosemary honey + essential oil of rosmarinus officinale (verbenon) + essential oil of thymus vulgaris (linalool) – to be taken internally.

Emphysema.
Propolis spray • Aroma-honey: eucalyptus honey + essential oil of eucalyptus globules + essential oil of rosmarinus officinalis (cineol 1.8).

Enterocolitis.
Propolis • Bee bread • Pollen • Aroma-honey: thyme honey + essential oil of thymus vulgaris (linalol) + essential oil of melaleuca alternifolia + essential oil of origanum majorana.

Erythema/Rash.
Lavender propo-honey applied directly to the skin • Aroma-honey: lavender honey + essential oil of lavandula angustifolia (vera) applied directly to the skin.

Exhaustion.
Pollen • Royal jelly • Aroma-honey: rosemary honey + essential oils of rosmarinus officinalis (camphor), satureja montana and chamaemelum nobile.

'Flu.
Propolis • Aroma-honey: thyme or sweet-chestnut honey + essential oil

of ravensara aromatica + essential oil of mentha piperata + essential oil of laurus nobilis.

Fungal Infections.
Skin infections: propolis tincture • Vaginal infections: Pessaries made up of propolis + essential oil of cinnamomum camphora • Infections of the digestive system or blood (candida albicans): propolis, aroma-honey: thyme honey + essential oil of thymus vulgaris (thujanol) + essential oil of cymbopogon martinii (palmarosa).

Furunculosis (Internal Treatment).
Propolis • Aroma-honey: thyme honey + essential oil of thymus (geraniol) + essential oil of melaleuca alternifolia + essential oil of ravensara aromatica.

Gall Stones.
This is in addition to medical treatment • Aroma-honey: rosemary honey + essential oil of juniperus communis (terpineol) + essential oil of rosmarinus officinalis (verbenon acetate) + essential oil of pinus mugo + essential oil of anetum graveolens OR: Aroma-honey: lemon blossom honey + essential oil of citrus limon + essential oil of juniperus communis (terpineol).

Gastralgia.
Propolis • Aroma-honey: multi-floral mountain honey + essential oil of mentha piperata + essential oil of origanum majorana + essential oil of cannabis sativa.

Gastritis.
Propolis • Bee bread • Aroma-honey: thyme or wild thyme honey + essential oil of acorus calamus asaroniferum + essential oil of mentha piperata.

Gastro-duodenal Ulcer (Helicobacter Pylori).
Propolis • Propolis tincture • Manuka honey • Aroma-honey: rosemary honey + essential oil of rosmarinus officinalis (verbenon) + essential oil of ocimum basilicum basilicum + essential oil of mentha piperata.

ALPHABETICAL LISTING OF AILMENTS

Gastro-intestinal Fermentation and/or Flatulence.
Bee bread • Propolis • Pollen • Aroma-honey: thyme honey + essential oil of mentha piperata + essential oil of thymus vulgaris (linalool) + essential oil of laurus nobilis.

General Fatigue and Chronic Fatigue.
Pollen • Bee bread • Royal jelly • Aroma-honey: floral mountain honey + essential oil of mentha piperata + essential oil of pinus sylvester OR: Aroma-honey: thyme honey + essential oil of Artemisia dracunculus + essential oil of ocimum basilicum basilicum + essential oil of helichrisum italicum.

Gingivitis.
Propolis tincture • Propolis gumdrops.

Gout (see also Uric Acid).
Aroma-honey: heather honey + essential oil of mentha piperata + + essential oil of birch + essential oil of rosmarinus officinalis (verbenon) • Apipuncture - micro-stinging administered by a specialist practitioner.

Gumboil (with or without Abscess).
Propolis tincture • Aroma-honey: thyme honey + essential oil of thymus (geraniol) + essential oil of melaleuca alternifolia + essential oil of Eugenia caryophyllus.

Hair Loss.
Acacia or lavender honey + royal jelly massaged into the scalp • Pollen.

Hay Fever – see under Allergies.

High Blood Pressure.
Lavender honey, orange blossom honey, rosemary honey, or lime blossom honey • Aroma-honey: rosemary honey + essential oil of rosmarinus officinalis camphoriferum (low concentration, less than 0.5%) + essential oil of alium sativum OR: Aroma-honey: rosemary honey + essential oil of rosmarinus officinalis cineol 1.8 + essential

oil of helichrisum italicum + essential oil of cupressus sempervirens. OR: Aroma-honey: orange blossom honey + essential oil of citrus aurantium aurantium neroli bigarade + essential oil of citrus reticulate mandarin peel + essential oil of citrus limon lemon peel.

Hoarseness.

Propolis spray
Miel de Sapin* honey
Aroma-honey: Miel de Sapin* honey + essential oil of rosmarinus officinalis (cineol 1.8) + essential oil of pinus sylvester

Hot Flushes.

Royal jelly
Pollen
Aroma-honey: hawthorn honey + essential oil of salvia officinalis sage + essential oil of ravensara anisata + essential oil of cupressus sempervirens (leaves)

Indigestion.
Propolis • Aroma-honey: multi-floral mountain honey + essential oil of mentha piperata + essential oil of origanum majorana + essential oil of rosmarinus officinalis (verbenon) OR: Aroma-honey: thyme or wild-thyme honey + essential oil of acorus calamus asaroniferum + essential oil of mentha piperata + essential oil of anethum graveolens.

Infections due to Staphylococcus Aureus.
Propolis • Aroma-honey: thyme honey + essential oil of melaleuca alternifolia + essential oil of ravensara aromatica + essential oil of thymus vulgaris (thymol) + essential oil of rosmarinus officinalis (verbenon).

Immune Deficiency.
Royal jelly • Pollen • Propolis • Aroma-honey: multi-floral mountain honey + essential oil of ravensara aromatica + essential oil of cupressus sempervirens + essential oil of thymus vulgaris (thymol) + essential oil

of laurus nobilis. In extreme and chronic cases: Apipuncture administered via micro-stings by a specialist practitioner.

Insomnia.

Lavender honey or orange blossom honey or lime blossom honey or lemon blossom honey • Aroma-honey: lavender honey + essential oil of lavandula angustifolia (vera) + essential oil of archangelica roots. OR: Aroma-honey: orange blossom honey + essential oil of chamaemelum nobilis + essential oil of matricaria recutita + essential oil of citrus aurantium bergamia peel.

Kidney Stones.
This is in addition to medical treatment.

Aroma-honey: heather honey + essential oil of juniperus communis (terpineol) + essential oil of agathosma betulina + essential oil of acorus calamus asaroniferum (long-term usage not recommended).

Laryngitis.

Lavender honey, thyme honey, eucalyptus honey or Miel de Sapin* honey • Propolis tincture • Propo-honey: above honeys + propolis • Aroma-honey: above honeys + essential oil of pinus pinaster + essential oil of thymus vulgaris (geraniol).

Leucorrhoea (Vaginal Discharge).

Propolis pessaries • Pessaries made up of propolis + essential oil of salvia sclarea + essential oil of salvia officinalis.

Liver Complaints.

Pollen • Bee bread • Propo-honey from rosemary honey • Aroma-honey: rosemary honey + essential oil of rosmarinus officinalis (verbenon) + essential oil of mentha piperata + essential oil of daucus carota.

Liver Failure.

Propolis • Bee bread • Aroma-honey: rosemary honey + essential oil of rosmarinus officinalis (camphor) + essential oil of anethum graveolens + essential oil of citrus lemon (peel).

Loss of Appetite.
Royal jelly • Pollen • Bee bread.

Low Blood Pressure.
Miel de Sapin* honey • Pollen • Bee bread • Royal jelly • Aroma-honey: Miel de Sapin* honey + essential oil of pinus sylvestris + essential oil of satureja montana + essential oil of mentha piperata. OR: Aroma-honey: rosemary honey + essential oil of rosmarinus officinalis camphoriferum + essential oil of pinus sylvestris + essential oil of mentha piperata.

Lupus.
Lavender honey - local application • Lavender propo-honey - local application • Aroma-honey: lavender honey + essential oil of angustifolia (vera) + essential oil of lavandula spica (local application). Propolis.

Lymph Node Diseases and Lymphadenopathy.
Propolis • Bee bread • Aroma-honey: mountain multi-floral honey + essential oils of cupressus sempervirens, ravensara aromatica, aniba roseodora, cymbopogon martinii (palmarosa).

Lymphatic (Blood Flow Decongestant).
Aroma-honey: lavender honey + essential oil of cupressus sempervirens + essential oil of pinus laricio + essential oil of myrtus communis myrtenylacetatiferum (local application) • Royal jelly.

Menopause.
Pollen • Royal jelly • Aroma-honey: multi-floral honey + essential oil of ravensara anisata + essential oil of salvia officinalis + essential oil of cupressus sempervirens. OR: Aroma-honey: lavender honey + essential oil of ravensara anisata + essential oil of salvia sclarea + essential oil of pimpinella anisum.

Metritis.
Propolis pessaries • Pessaries made up of propolis + essential oil of angustifolia (vera).

Migraine.

Aroma-honey: rosemary honey + essential oil of betula alleghaniensis
If the migraine is of hepatic and/or digestive origin:-
Aroma-honey: multi-floral mountain honey + essential oil of mentha piperata + essential oil of ocimum basilicum basilicum + essential oil of Artemisia draconculus.

Mouth Ulcers.

Thyme honey • Propo-honey with thyme honey • Alcoholic tincture of propolis • Aroma-honey: thyme honey + essential oils of ravensara aromatica, mentha piperata and ocimum basilicum basilicum.

Multiple Sclerosis.

Apipuncture administered by a specialist practitioner • Royal jelly • Aroma-honey: multi-flower honey from the mountains + essential oil of laurus nobilis + essential oil of cistus ladaniferus pineniferum.

Nephritis.

Aroma-honey: heather honey + essential oil of Artemisia dracunculus + essential oil of anethum graveolens + essential oil of juniperus communis (o.p. berries) • Pollen • Bee bread.

Nervous Conditions and Depression.

Lime blossom honey • Royal jelly • Aroma-honey: lime blossom honey + essential oil of chamaemelum nobile + essential oil of cannabis sativa + essential oil of hypericum perforatum.

Neuralgia.

Aroma-honey: multi-floral mountain honey + essential oil of gaultheria fragrantissima + essential oil of mentha piperata + essential oil of origanum marjorana • Royal jelly

Osteoarthritis.

Apipuncture administered by a specialist practitioner • Propolis • Pollen
Aroma-honey: rosemary honey + essential oils of rosmarinus (verbenon acetate), satureoid thymus and origanum marjorana.

Ovarian Inflammation.
Pessaries made up of alcoholic propolis tincture + essential oil of cupressus sempervirens + essential oil of eucalyptus citriodora + essential oil of ravensara anisata. OR: Pessaries made up of alcoholic propolis tincture + essential oil of cupressus sempervirens + essential oil of salvia officinale.

Parkinson's Disease.
Apipuncture administered by a specialist practitioner.

Period Pains.
Royal jelly • Sweet chestnut honey • Aroma-honey: Sweet chestnut honey + essential oil of cupressus sempervirens + essential oil of salvia sclarea + essential oil of chamaemelum nobilis.

Piles.
Propolis suppositories + essential oil of cupressus sempervirens • Aroma-honey: Sweet chestnut or heather honey + essential oil of cupressus sempervirens + essential oil of melaleuca cajeputii.

Post-natal Depression.
Pollen • Royal jelly • Once breastfeeding has ceased: Aroma-honey: lemon blossom honey + essential oil of citrus limonum (peel) + essential oil of cinnamomum zeylanicum (bark) OR: Aroma-honey: lavender honey + essential oil of salvia officinalis + essential oil of rosmarinus officinalis (verbenon) + essential oil of Eugenia caryophylatta (clove).

Pregnancy.
Royal jelly • Mountain multi-floral honey, lavender honey, orange blossom honey, or lime blossom honey • The above honeys + royal jelly (1% concentration) massaged onto the belly after softening in a bain-marie (max 35°C) for the prevention of stretch marks.

Pressure Sores.
Lavender honey, sweet chestnut honey, rosemary honey, thyme honey or multi-floral mountain honey applied directly to the skin • Propo-honey from any of the above, applied directly to the skin • Apipuncture via

micro-stings administered by a specialist practitioner.

Prostatitis.
Pollen • Propolis • Bee bread • Aroma-honey: thyme or heather honey + essential oil of cupressus sempervirens + essential oil of mentha piperata + essential oil of eucalyptus polybractea cryptonifera + essential oil of pinus laricio.

Prurigo (Dermatitis).
Lavender honey applied locally • Aroma-honey: lavender honey + essential oil of angustifolia (vera) applied locally • Lavender propohoney applied locally.

Rash (See also Allergies).
Aroma-honey: lavender honey + essential oil of angustifolia (vera) in topical application.

Rheumatic Fever.
Apipuncture administered by a specialist practitioner • Aroma-honey: thyme honey + essential oil of thymus vulgaris (linalool) + essential oil of ravensara aromatica + essential oil of citrus aurantium (leaves).

Rheumatism.
Propolis • Apipuncture administered by a specialist practitioner • Aroma-honey: rosemary honey + essential oil of rosmarinus officinalis (verbenon) + essential oil of laurus nobilis + essential oil of juniperus communis (berries) + essential oil of origanum majorana.

Rheumatoid Arthritis.
Propolis • Apipuncture administered by a specialist practitioner • Aroma-honey: thyme or rosemary honey + essential oil of ocimum basilicum basilicum + essential oil of eucalyptus citriodora + essential oil of helichrysum italicum + essential oil of laurus nobilis.

Rickets.
Royal jelly • Pollen • Bee larvae • Bee bread • Honey + royal jelly + bee bread.

Roundworm.
Propo-honey • Propolis • Aroma-honey: mountain multi-floral honey or thyme honey + essential oils of allium sativum, melaleuca alternifolia and thymus vulgaris (linalool).

Sciatica.
Apipuncture administered by a specialist practitioner.

Sinusitis.
Alcoholic tincture of propolis • Aroma-honey: rosemary honey + essential oil of rosmarinus (cineol 1.8) + essential oil of helichrysum italicum + essential oil of origanum marjorana (in case of acute sinusitis, add essential oil of pinus sylvestris).

Sore Throat (Pharyngitis).
Propolis tincture (local application) • Propolis • Aroma-honey: eucalyptus or thyme or lavender honey + essential oil of eucalyptus globulus + essential oil of rosmarinus (1.8 cineol) + essential oil of ravensara aromatica + essential oil of thymus vulgaris (thujanol).

Stomatitis.
Propolis • Alcoholic tincture of propolis • Aroma-honey: thyme honey + essential oil of thymus vulgaris (linalol) + essential oil of thymus vulgaris (thujanol).

Stress.
Royal jelly • Pollen • Lavender honey.

Tapeworm.
Propo-honey • Propolis • Aroma-honey: thyme honey or multi-flower mountain honey + essential oil of allium sativum + essential oil of thymus vulgaris (linalool) + essential oil of thymus vulgaris (thujanol)

Tonsilitis.
Lavender honey • Propolis alcohol tincture • Propo-honey with lavender honey • Propo-aroma-honey: propolis tincture + thyme honey + essential oil of thymus vulgaris (either geraniol or linalool).

Threadworms.

Propo-honey • Propolis • Aroma-honey: multi-floral mountain honey or thyme honey + essential oil of allium sativum + essential oil of thymus vulgaris (thujanol).

Thrombosis.

Aroma-honey: lavender honey or sweet chestnut honey + essential oil of angustifolia (vera) + essential oil of cupressus sempervirens, applied locally • Apipuncture administered as micro-puncture by a specialist practitioner • Bee bread.

Tracheititis.

Mountain multi-flower honey, lavender honey, Miel de Sapin* honey or eucalyptus honey • Propolis tincture • Propo-honey made from the abovementioned honeys • Aroma-honey: eucalyptus honey + essential oil of eucalyptus radiata + essential oil of eucalyptus smitii OR: Aroma-honey: Miel de Sapin* honey + essential oil of cupressus sempervirens + essential oil of myrtus communis (cineol 1.8) + essential oil of eucalyptus radiata.

Tuberculosis.

In addition to medical treatment:

Bee bread • Propolis • Aroma-honey: Miel de Sapin* honey + essential oil of cupressus sempervirens + essential oil of ravensara aromatica + essential oil of myrtus communis (cineol 1.8) + essential oil of laurus nobilis.

Uric acid

Propo-aroma-honey: heather honey + Alcoholic tincture of propolis + essential oils of betula alba, rosmarinus officinalis (verbenon).

Vaginitis (Infectious).

Pessaries made up of alcoholic propolis tincture + essential oil of melaleuca alternifolia + essential oil of thymus vulgaris (linalool).

Varicose Veins.

Aroma-honey: mountain multi-floral honey + essential oil of

helichrysum italicum + essential oil of melaleuca quinquinerva + essential oil of cupressus sempervirens • The following to be applied overnight: Aroma-honey: mountain multi-floral honey + essential oil of cupressus sempervirens + essential oil of lavandula angustifolia (vera).

Vomiting (Motion Sickness).

Aroma-honey: mountain multi-floral honey + essential oil of mentha piperata.

Weight Loss (Anorexia).

Pollen • Royal jelly • Bee bread • Rosemary honey.

Whitlow.

Aroma-honey: thyme honey + essential oil of melaleuca alternifolia + essential oil of angustifolia (vera) applied locally.

Worms.

Propo-honey • Propolis • Aroma-honey: mountain multi-floral honey or thyme honey + essential oil of allium sativum + essential oil of thymus vulgaris (linalool) + essential oil of thymus vulgaris (thujanol). OR: Aroma-honey: honey + essential oils of bergamot, eucalyptus and lavender.

ALPHABETICAL LISTING OF AILMENTS

DESCRIPTION OF THE HEALING BEE
(PUBLISHED IN THE ORIGINAL EDITION)

Roch Domerego is one of the most eminent specialists in the field of apitherapy, that is to say the science of "healing through the use of bee products", which is a mixture of traditional and modern thinking which reconciles man with nature. In this fascinating book he takes us on a voyage of discovery into a harmonious world from which we have a lot to learn.

It has always been common knowledge that products from the hive are good for human health, and today we regard these old remedies from our grandparents' time with benevolent condescension. However, recent scientific research has demonstrated that the various substances manufactured by honeybees, alongside endless combinations with plant products, are indeed virtual medicines, with properties superior to those of chemical remedies, and without any adverse side effects or costly outlay. Roch Domerego draws our attention to the ocean of hope offered by 'green medicine' for the wellbeing of tablet-happy Westerners, as well as for the survival of people in poor countries.

For the first time, he also reveals the fruit of his many years' experience: practical recipes to treat over a hundred pathologies.

Here at last we can find out how to look after our health simply, naturally… and efficiently.

Roch Domerego is a Naturotherapist and a university professor; he is vice-president of the Apitherapy Commission within Apimondia (the central body for beekeepers from all over the world). He lives in Brussels.

www.ingramcontent.com/pod-product-compliance
Lightning Source LLC
Chambersburg PA
CBHW080546170426
43195CB00016B/2700